# The
# CANCER
# Effect

# The CANCER Effect

by
CLAUDIA BRETZING

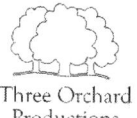

Three Orchard
Productions

The Cancer Effect

Copyright © 2016 by Claudia Bretzing. All rights reserved. No part of this publication may be reproduced, distributed, or transmitted in any form or by any means, including photocopying, recording, or other electronic or mechanical methods, without the prior written permission of the publisher, except in the case of brief quotations embodied in critical reviews and certain other noncommercial uses permitted by copyright law. For permission requests, write to the publisher, at the address below.

Three Orchard Productions
4435 E. Broadway Road, Suite 6
Mesa, Arizona 85206

Cover Art by Abigail E. Fowkes
abbiefowkes.art@gmail.com

Author: Claudia Bretzing
cabretzing@gmail.com
www.TheCancerEffect.com

Disclaimer: The information and experiences in this book are not intended to replace any advice, medical or otherwise, and are not to be used or relied on for any diagnostic or treatment purposes. The author and/or publisher do not endorse or disclaim specifically any test, treatment, procedure or course of action mentioned in this book. The reader should always consult his/her health care provider before making any health care decisions or for guidance about any health-related condition. The author and/or publisher expressly disclaim responsibility, and shall have no liability, for any damages, loss, injury, or liability whatsoever suffered as a result of the reader's reliance on the information contained in this book.

Some names and identifying details have been changed to protect the privacy of individuals.

ISBN 0-9969313-6-8
ISBN 978-0-9969313-6-6

Printed in the United States of America

"I am not afraid of storms,
for I am learning how to sail my ship."

Louisa May Alcott, *Little Women*

# **DEDICATION**

This book is dedicated to anyone
who has heard the words, "It's cancer,"
and to all their companions on the journey,
who endured the agony of watching.

And to Randy, my dear husband,
who held my hand every step of the way.

# TABLE OF CONTENTS

| | |
|---|---|
| Introduction | ix |
| THE DISCOVERY | 1 |
| COPING | 31 |
| SURGERY | 53 |
| THE FIRST CHEMO | 89 |
| THE NEW PLAN | 113 |
| HAIR TODAY, GONE TOMORROW | 135 |
| UNDAUNTED | 153 |
| THE FINAL CHEMO | 179 |
| MY NEVER ENDING STORY | 185 |
| NEW CHALLENGES | 201 |
| THE TROUBLE WITH DRUGS | 213 |
| INSTEAD, I HAVE CURLS | 227 |
| HELP IN HEALING | 237 |
| THE FEAR SYNDROME | 253 |
| MORE THAN JUST SURVIVING | 263 |
| Book Club Discussion Questions | 290 |
| Acknowledgements | 293 |
| Contact the Author | 298 |

# INTRODUCTION

I am a cancer survivor.

What does it mean to survive? A simple dictionary definition would be "to live through a life-threatening experience". I am here to say I survived the necessary treatments designed to rid my body of cancer cells. However, my cancer journey has taught me that surviving encompasses so much more. The German philosopher Friedrich Nietzsche said, "To live is to suffer. To survive is to find some meaning in the suffering."

This book took me six years to write because I needed that long to understand surviving. When I learned I had breast cancer, being cured was my only objective and the reason I searched for a doctor and treatment plan that I could trust.

There was nothing that could have sufficiently prepared me for the physical crusade ahead, but science had a plan. Millions of dollars and years of study and research have been expended to assist a cancer patient in the quest to physically survive. When diagnosed with cancer, the primary focus is to ensure the enemy is eliminated and the patient lives.

Physically surviving took all my time and energy, and after eight months, I finally achieved my goal. I thought I had arrived and was finished, only to find I faced another obstacle, one I was not expecting.

Facing side effects from months of chemotherapy, the fear of cancer returning and invading other areas of my body and struggling to discover my new normal sent me spiraling. Just as I floundered when I was first diagnosed with cancer, I lacked direction trying to survive emotionally. I wasn't prepared and emotional survival could not be accomplished with a clear-cut treatment plan. To be complete again, I would need to conquer the challenges of emotionally surviving cancer and its effects.

One breast cancer survivor described it as a race. When we all began this journey, our eyes were on the finish line and when our physical bodies reached that point, which symbolized the end of treatment, we realized that our emotions were back at the starting line, where we had left them. We didn't have the strength at the time to carry them with us, or even realize they existed. It was all we could do to survive the physical torments of chemotherapy and radiation. Now we had to go back and bring our emotional selves along to the finish.

When I began writing this book, I wrote with the intention of helping others who were diagnosed with cancer. That is still my hope, but writing has come with an unexpected bonus. As I allowed myself to gradually open and scrutinize my complex emotions, I achieved personal healing. When I started this book, I expected the last chapter to be The Final Chemo, but when this day ended, I realized there was more story that needed to be told. The number of chapters far exceeded my expectations as I discovered the effects of cancer extend miles beyond my first vision of the journey. Each step forward, though slow and often plodding, was a necessary stride towards learning and self-discovery.

Each person must make a choice when faced with life's challenges. We can either strive to find the lessons and opportunities for growth, or we can merely survive the best we can and move on after the storm, never bothering to clean up the clutter. It is easier to leave the mess, but infinitely better to pick through the rubble and come face to face with reality. With newly acquired knowledge, it is then our responsibility to share it and calm the storm for the next victim.

I learned that one must be careful when digging through the rubble to not get caught in the muck. At times, I found I was stagnating while going through this process and had to pull myself up by my boot straps and get moving again. Discovering how to leave the past behind without forgetting the experience and valuable lessons was vital to my recovery. I needed to eliminate the constant fear that one small cancer cell survived treatment and would someday return to interrupt my life. That is a possibility, but faith and fear cannot co-exist.

It is a tricky process to move forward after dealing with a life-threatening disease. True, my life would forever be changed from my original course, but I couldn't keep making pit stops. I had to learn to constantly press ahead.

Allowing others to see me from the inside out isn't comfortable, but if my story brings a smile to your face or an occasional tear, it has been worth it. If my words help you know you aren't alone in this journey, and if you find hope and courage in these pages, I have succeeded in more than just surviving.

This book has a last page, but my story does not. It continues as I keep learning lessons about surviving cancer. I don't expect the road ahead to be free of struggles and surprises, but I no longer fear, and I'm comfortable with what I have become through this process. I am better equipped to face whatever the future may hold. Yes, I'm a survivor, and even if my battle resumes, I'm still victorious, because I learned to believe, to have faith, and to trust in God.

*July 11, 2009*

*Dear Journal,*

*It has been four days since I learned I had cancer. I have not been able to write as I can't find the words to describe my feelings. In the past, I've never had a problem pinpointing my emotions and the course I should take. I feel like someone has taken my mind and put it in a blender, making it impossible to identify any one feeling. As a result, I've been trying to keep busy and not dwell on the reality of my situation.*

*I'm pretty certain no one suspects the degree of my perplexity at this time, as I'm doing a pretty good job of portraying optimism, a role I play fairly well.*

# THE DISCOVERY

I didn't know how long I had been staring at the same page in the tattered magazine I was holding. My thoughts were not on the small waiting room or the stiff pink paper gown I was wearing. I was thinking about my mother who once had a lump in her breast, her surgery, and the benign results. Surely that would be the worst I would have to endure. I had to stay positive. That was my nature.

My thoughts briefly took me back to earlier that morning when I was getting ready for this mammogram. My mind was more on what I planned to accomplish after what I considered to be a routine visit than on the exam itself. When I walked through those doors, I anticipated the usual procedure of undressing from the waist up, the imaging, redressing, and exiting unruffled through those same doors. Checking the appointment off my list, I would be free to complete the rest of my plans for the day.

I must admit I did have some trepidation, due to the unusual change I had noticed on the surface of my breast. When did I notice it? I don't remember. It finally motivated me to make an appointment with my nurse practitioner, whose recommendation brought me to this point, only eleven months since my last mammogram. Eleven months. What could possibly change in just eleven months? That alone gave me some comfort and reassurance.

The standard mammogram was over, but I was still sitting in this grim room draped in the pink gown. Instead of being released to the cubicle to retrieve my clothing, I was asked to sit and wait because more imaging was required. Apparently, my feigned confidence could not deceive modern science. The monster camera must have sighted something unusual.

I had effectively brushed my worries aside for months and now I was being forced to face them. I felt jittery and wished I could be anywhere but on this hard chair. It was a hot summer day outside, but suspicions arising from the mammogram sent chills throughout my body. Surely this was just a cautious check to make sure all was well. My mind kept racing in circles between feeble attempts to think positive and the realization that something might be wrong.

Again, I reasoned that all would turn out all right, just as it had with my mom. I felt some degree of reassurance knowing that I could always check "No" to the question, "Is there a history of cancer in your family?" Not one member of my immediate family had ever had cancer.

If I were to be honest with myself, however, I had to face the haunting fact that I actually didn't know anything about my birth father's side of the family. I remember seeing him once but knew little about the circumstances that surrounded him. He was a stranger and his absence in my life led to half my genetic make-up being a mystery, a fact that might make a difference. I also needed to remember that not everyone who gets cancer has a genetic predisposition for it, either.

My thoughts were abruptly interrupted by the gentle voice of the lab technician. They were ready to begin my ultrasound. She tried to engage in small talk as we solemnly walked into a room I previously never had reason to enter—the room where my nightmare began.

Then again, was that sterile, unfriendly room really the beginning? As a second-grade teacher, I teach my students the simple concept that every story has a beginning, a middle, and an end. But my story doesn't seem so simple—I don't know when everything began. Microscopic cancer cells were multiplying and invading healthy tissue long before the outward symptoms appeared. I innocently carried on with my life, oblivious to the eventual betrayal I would experience.

My story doesn't have an ending either, another rule of writing I choose to ignore. When I began my cancer journey, I was confident there would be an end and that is what got me through the worst days. But as anyone who has traveled the cancer road knows, it never really ends, unless you don't survive.

Even though I have no idea when my feet were planted on a road I never planned to travel, I do need to start this story somewhere. It seems natural to begin during my favorite time of year, about six months before the cancer effect turned my world upside down and inside out.

The Christmas of 2008 was as busy and happy a time as I can remember. Our son Doug had recently returned from two years in Taiwan as a missionary for our church. All five of his siblings, their spouses, and a host of nieces and nephews would be at our home for the holidays—a total of nineteen in all. I wanted everything to be perfect for my family, which meant hours of planning and preparation. Cherished Christmas traditions had evolved through the years with extensive decorating both inside and out, gingerbread houses, appealing desserts, games, and the music of the season. It was a deeply joyful time, free of any worries or regard for subtle changes in my body that I chose to ignore, or take precious time to think about.

After the New Year celebrations, I embarked upon my daily routine of teaching second grade. January was hectic with our study of penguins and whales and preparations for parent teacher conferences. Had I noticed that the nipple on my left breast was inverted? If I did I paid it little, if any consideration. I recall thinking at one point that perhaps it was just a normal sign of an aging body. I felt great and I wasn't concerned. My life was crowded with many things to do and many events, including the birth of our eighth grandchild, a handsome little boy. Life could not be sweeter.

In March, we traveled to Utah to join family members for the wedding of our son, Doug, and his sweet bride, Whitney. That was my first memory of thinking more than a few seconds about the change in my body. As I got in the shower one morning, I glanced down and noticed the nipple on my left breast seemed more inverted than I previously remembered. Was I just imagining it? For the first time, I checked for a lump but didn't feel anything and dismissed any nagging worries since my mammogram last summer was unremarkable. It would be time for my yearly check-up this coming July, so I made a mental note to call and make an appointment when I got home. I recalled that appointments are usually booked out three months in advance so I shouldn't delay. The matter concerned me so little that I didn't even mention it to anyone.

April and May were nothing but a blur. Those are two very hectic months for a school teacher, crammed with testing and all other necessary activities to tie up the end of the school year. I was also preparing to teach summer school the entire month of June. Had I followed up on my mental reminder to make my yearly appointment? Not yet, and it was getting more difficult to ignore the nagging feeling that I should take care of the matter. As it was now, I wouldn't be able to get in until the end of the summer, or worse, the beginning of the next school year. I even considered waiting until I had time off in December. After all, these yearly exams always came out fine and waiting a few more months shouldn't make any difference.

How long does it take to make a phone call? Probably two minutes if you aren't placed on hold. While I was too busy to take time out of my hectic schedule, cancer cells continued to quietly divide and spread, invading lymph nodes as well as my left breast.

The last three days of May found my husband Randy and I involved in a youth activity for our church. The plans were to re-enact the days of the pioneers and the challenges they faced as they trekked through primitive, unsettled land to go west. The youth were divided into families of ten with a Ma and Pa to guide them. Randy and I were asked to be a Ma and Pa of such a group and since we had done it before when our son was in high school, we were excited to participate again. This time our youngest daughter, Brittany, would be going. The committee that organized this trek thought of everything from renting wooden handcarts and choosing the rocky trail we would traverse, to the mundane food we would eat. Everyone dressed in authentic pioneer clothing and left all technology, from cell phones to flashlights, behind.

The first day was designed to be the most difficult as we walked and pushed a handcart with all our provisions for twenty miles through the rough mountain terrain near Prescott, Arizona. The second and third days were directed toward more engaging activities such as pioneer games, killing and plucking a chicken for our dinner, and attending inspiring campfire programs.

During the first day of our long trek I was surprised to find I did not have the strength and endurance I expected. We were required to push loaded handcarts up steep, rocky inclines, as well as hike for hours. Starting after a healthy breakfast of oranges, granola, and rolls, we walked for a short distance on relatively flat ground. Everyone was in good spirits, displaying the energy of youth, most having no idea what was ahead. When we reached the base of the trail that led up a mountain, we stared in disbelief at what would be required of our rickety wooden handcarts, not to mention our own feet. The beginning of the trail was doable, but when we looked ahead at what was in store, the task seemed ludicrous. The trail wasn't suitable for a four-wheel drive truck, much less a two-wheeled handcart powered by humans.

As we pushed and pulled over huge craggy boulders and through thick beds of sand, our endurance and enthusiasm for the task waned. Being the Ma of our little family, I was expected to maintain a cheerful attitude and encourage those who struggled. By evening, Hunter, one of the boys in our group, kept falling behind, so I decided to stay back with him while the rest kept up their slow but steady pace.

As we trudged along watching other families pass, I became more concerned about Hunter. I could tell that he was sinking fast—he was dizzy and acting disoriented. We were not allowed to carry food, and our water supply was on the handcart, undoubtedly a mile away by now. This young man was my responsibility, yet I wasn't carrying anything that could help him.

We were breathing the dust of the last handcart when a lone boy joined us out of nowhere. He was carrying a backpack, an obvious infraction of the guidelines set for the trek. As I explained my concern for Hunter and his diminishing energy, this young man sprang into action. It was clear he was not a newcomer to outdoor survival when he pulled out a can of beans, opened them, and started feeding Hunter.

It didn't take long to see marked improvement in Hunter's appearance, filling me with relief and gratitude. Our rescuer had broken the rules of the trek, but not the rules of common sense. Lucky for us he had come prepared. As we rested and visited before resuming the hike, I looked with awe at our angel in disguise and was thankful he had made the choice to plan for an emergency. That night he was my hero.

He stayed with us, making sure we were all right until one of the adult leaders on horseback rode up to check our progress, or lack of it. After explaining the difficulty Hunter was experiencing, he was taken in a vehicle the rest of the way. I was left to finish the climb. My hero had disappeared, and though I looked for him, I never saw him again.

By this point the sun had gone down, and the chances of reuniting with my family were slim. Fortunately, I wasn't alone. I shared the trail with a few others who had lagged behind and we stumbled along together, finally catching up to a handcart group that was resting. At least now we had some light to guide our steps since they had lanterns. We continued to walk for hours in silence, except for all the complaining that was rolling through my mind. It was hard to maintain a positive attitude with aching feet, lack of nourishment, and no end in sight.

Reaching the first night's camp at 3:00 a.m., I collapsed from an exhaustion I had never experienced before. Turning down the broth and hard roll I was offered, I found my sleeping bag and searched for the least rocky spot of ground I could find. Since the flat stretches of land were already occupied, I settled for a spot on a slight incline, away from most of our group. It was better that my family didn't observe my current state of mind. My ability to be upbeat was long gone, having vanished several miles back. I knew getting some sleep would improve my attitude as well as my aching body, even if it would only be for a few hours. As I lay on the hard ground trying to fall asleep, I wondered why I was having such a tough time this year. Being three years older than the last experience shouldn't make that much difference.

As tired as I was, I never slept that short night. I found if I didn't keep my legs perfectly straight, I would experience painful muscle spasms. Every time I drifted off to sleep, my legs would relax and bend, awakening me with a jerk. My biggest concern as I stared into the black night was how I would lead my little pioneer family the next day with little sleep and no energy. From past experience, I knew every moment would be filled with activities and resting would be out of the question. I became increasingly more frustrated at my inability to sleep, which of course added to my dilemma. I was near the breaking point.

As I lay there completely exhausted, alone in my thoughts, I finally decided to pray for the ability to not just endure the rest of this trip, but endure it well. I definitely needed divine help to face the next day and all that would be required of me. Despite my own physical distress, I wanted to appear cheerful and enthusiastic. My attitude would greatly affect those of my group. With that resolve, I watched the dreaded signs of early dawn approach, trying to relax as much as possible on the rocky terrain beneath my sleeping bag.

After eating a miserable breakfast of cornmeal with no milk, our little company hiked for several more miles before entering a clearing where we set up camp. That accomplished, we were directed to the various planned activities designed to give us a taste of pioneer life. By evening, I was leading a small group of my family in preparing the first decent meal of the trek. It included the chicken the youth had killed and plucked earlier that day, combined with vegetables to make a chicken stew. It turned out the only edible part of the long-awaited feast were the vegetables as the chicken was too tough to eat. The meal was saved by some bread dough which we fried into scones, complimented by the butter and honey we found in our supplies. I was feeding ten hungry teenagers, so it didn't take long to devour our allotted rations.

I was never more relieved to have night come with the opportunity to finally sleep. I fell asleep quickly, only to awaken a few hours later, shaking from the drastic drop in temperature. My light sleeping bag wasn't made for extreme weather, and I spent another restless night trying to overcome the cold and the intermittent drizzling rain.

It was through divine intervention and a large dose of will power that I completed the pioneer trek of 2009. I had faced challenges that tested even the younger members of our group, and I was fifty-eight years old, a few years past my prime. After it was over, I remarked to my husband Randy, "Now I know I can do really hard things."

Despite the hardships, or because of them, it was one of the best experiences of my life. Not even imagining I had cancer at the time of this trek, I was unknowingly being prepared to face the hardest uphill climb of my life. I had never been so physically challenged before and the lessons I learned about my ability to endure pain and suffering helped me through some very difficult moments ahead. I have no doubt that God knows what is coming and he provides us with learning experiences to get our minds and hearts ready. If we are wise, we recognize we are being tutored, and pay close attention.

The second week of June was when I finally called to make an appointment for my yearly female physical. I'm not sure what motivated me to pick up the phone, except my noisy conscience reminding me of its importance. I also knew that unless I made an appointment, the office wouldn't refill my prescription for estrogen which I had been taking since my hysterectomy in 2001. When I called, I was amazed there was an opening for the following Wednesday afternoon. I don't look forward to these appointments and since I wasn't expecting to get one so soon, I almost turned it down. Not being able to come up with a good reason, I accepted the time offered, glad to check one more item off my "to do" list for the summer.

The office was familiar as I had used this group for my check-ups for several years, even after my favorite doctor left. Since I had no real issues or problems, I was fine going to the nurse practitioner, Amber. During the exam, she didn't comment on the change in my breast until I finally pointed it out to her. She seemed interested, but not concerned, and suggested I schedule a mammogram right away. My chart indicated that it had been eleven months since my last mammogram and I knew my insurance only covered yearly visits. She assured me that her referral would be diagnostic which would eliminate that issue. I made the appointment for the following Friday.

In my mind the upcoming appointment wasn't worth any more consideration than jotting it on my calendar. What anxiety I had over the change in my breast had been dissipated by my nurse practitioner who didn't seem too worried even after I pointed it out. I reasoned she was just being cautious by ordering a mammogram a few weeks early. It all seemed routine to me and I spent the subsequent days focused on teaching summer school and preparing for our family trip to Utah, scheduled for the first of July.

The day of the mammogram appointment came quickly and I got ready like any other morning. Little did I know my world was about to be turned upside down. I would soon begin a journey for which no one can prepare, nor expect to take. How is it that one pivotal moment can change everything?

After being shown a small dressing room, I put on the pink paper gown and waited for my turn. I browsed through a magazine laying close by but couldn't settle on an article to read. I found it difficult to concentrate and was beginning to feel a little nervous, knowing there was a definite change in my left breast. I kept reminding myself there was probably nothing to worry about. I continued to try and locate an article worth reading to pass the time, but ended up staring at pages of meaningless advertisements. I've always hated waiting.

When it was finally my turn, I entered the room, accompanied by a pleasant technician. She gave me directions as she positioned me for each picture.

"Take a deep breath and hold it." Click. "Now breathe." Repeat.

I smiled thinking of friends who complained about having their breasts squished to the dimensions of a pancake. This was one occasion when not being well endowed was a blessing. After taking the usual pictures of each breast, I was asked to stay in the room for a few minutes. There was nothing unusual about that. In the past, the technician always checked to make sure she got all the needed angles before sending me off to get dressed. I was glad this was over and I could just wait like any other year for the call that would confirm all was normal. When she returned, she informed me that she would be taking a few more pictures of the left breast. Again I rationalized that they were just making sure nothing was amiss. It was good they were being thorough.

Upon completion of the mammogram, I quickly escaped the room intending to get dressed and continue with my day. However, my efforts to flee were thwarted when I was asked to remain in the gown. They wanted to do an ultrasound on my left breast.

Now I was worried. That request signaled something was discovered and would definitely result in this appointment lasting longer than I wanted. I picked up an old magazine lying on the chair next to me and started turning pages, trying desperately to distract my mind from the quickly gathering negative thoughts. As I stared blankly at the open page I had to wonder if my inverted nipple indicated a problem after all. Trying to grasp any possible positive thought floating out in space, I reminded myself that I had a perfectly normal mammogram less than a year ago.

The ultrasound took about twenty-five minutes. During this time, I was lying in an awkward position, listening to clicks of the machine, followed by the technician typing on the computer. No words were spoken, but my mind was jumping all over the place. *What was she seeing on the machine? Why was this additional imaging necessary? Maybe I should have come right in when I first noticed the inverted nipple.* And finally, but only once, I allowed myself to think, *What if it's cancer?*

I tried to focus on keeping my thoughts positive but didn't succeed very well. After taking multiple pictures of what seemed like every inch of my left breast, the technician finally said I could get dressed. My hopes of going home were dashed when she asked me to wait in a small room until someone came to talk with me. My protests went unvoiced but were echoing loudly inside. *What is there to talk about? What would you possibly need to tell me?*

I dressed quickly, relieved to be free of the scratchy gown. After a few minutes the same technician returned and apologized for asking me to get undressed again. They needed more pictures of a certain area. As I complied with her request, I suddenly wished Randy was by my side. I didn't like facing this unexpected uncertainty alone. I was doubting my previous optimism and wanted to be anywhere but at this imaging center taking more pictures and having a "talk".

As more ultrasound shots were taken, I tried to watch the screen this time to see if there was anything I could detect. Unfortunately, I didn't have the trained eye to decipher anything but a bunch of garbled shadows and I wondered how much training it took to develop the skills to read such imaging. After about ten minutes of additional scrutiny, the technician began rapidly typing what I thought was probably a report on the computer. As she finished, the uncomfortable silence was interrupted by the phone ringing. The technician spoke in hushed tones but there were enough words that came through to make me think, *I hope they aren't talking about me.* Then I heard her say, "Yes, she is sitting right here." My stomach lurched as I realized I was the topic of the present conversation and I was handed the phone.

On the other end of the line was a radiologist who introduced herself as a doctor. Without wasting words, she told me there was a suspicious spot on my breast that would need a biopsy. She stressed the importance of scheduling it right away. I politely thanked her for the unwanted information, not knowing what else to say. I just couldn't think clearly. When the shock wore off, I knew I would kick myself for not asking the countless questions that were already beginning to formulate. *How do I get a biopsy? Where do I go? What kind of suspicious spot, and was it just a spot, or was it a mass?*

I dressed quickly, anxious to escape the words I just heard. Maybe if I hurried I could outrun them, leaving them to rot in this dreadful place. As I left the building, I couldn't help but notice the strained stares of the two technicians who worked with me that day. They had been whispering together, stopping when they saw me come into view. The pitying looks in their eyes as they told me good-bye was not what I wanted to see. Maybe I was just imagining it. Maybe inwardly I knew the obvious.

As I drove home, I could hardly wait to talk about my appointment with Randy. He had the day off and I was glad I could share my worries and all that I had just experienced. What a disappointment to find him gone when I walked in our house. I called his cell phone and found he was shopping at Bass Pro Shop, a local sporting goods store. He sounded surprised when I told him I would be there in a few minutes. I like to shop, but usually pass when it comes to spending time looking at hunting and camping gear.

When I arrived, he was in good spirits and could hardly wait to show me the variety of different fudges available in one section of the store. He talked non-stop as we made our way past the women's T-shirts to the fudge counter. I tried to concentrate on helping him decide which ones we should buy, sampling a few to make our choices easier. How trivial to be talking about candy at a time like this. After purchasing the fudge, we walked for a while around the camping supplies, looking at nothing in particular and engaging in small talk.

Finally, I couldn't suppress my fears any longer, and shared with Randy what had happened at my appointment that morning. He was stunned and obviously shaken by the news, but our conversation remained positive.

I reminded him and myself, "You know my mom had a lump in her breast and they found it to be benign. We've never had cancer in our family, so I'm sure this is going to be the same."

"You're right. Most lumps are just that. Nothing to worry about," Randy assured me. I couldn't ignore the strain in his voice.

I don't think either of us wanted to think otherwise. We didn't discuss the other possibility, cancer, but it was a little demon that took residence in the back of our minds. Once that demon settles in, it remains, coming out whenever it feels like it to torment and rattle an otherwise quiet neighborhood.

As we arrived home, I absently placed the purchased fudge in the fridge and there it remained, untouched until it was thrown out, a grim reminder of the day we received the disturbing news. I can't believe we let ten dollars' worth of fudge go to waste.

My first inclination was not to mention any of this pending drama to my children until I received the results of the biopsy. Why worry them needlessly? I fantasized a scene in which I would tell them all that Dad and I had been through the last few weeks, with the outcome in my favor. It is always easier to talk about a trial after it has been resolved.

Five of my six children were grown and living away from home so it would be easy to remain quiet. Brittany, however was another story. She was my youngest and a very perceptive teenager. She could tell from my countenance that something was wrong that day. I tried to answer her probing questions honestly, so it didn't take her long to get the full story. After sharing the news with Brittany, I realized I should call and tell my other five children. I was going to need their support and prayers during this time of waiting. I was comfortable with this decision and immediately felt peace as I called and talked with each of them. Their positive words buoyed me up and I didn't feel alone. I knew I could face anything with the support of my family.

The next step was to try and think rationally about what I needed to accomplish first. I was told to schedule a biopsy but I had no idea where to go or how to proceed. That would have been a good question to ask the radiologist who emphasized the importance of acting quickly. I felt like I was in a maze with no idea which way to turn.

We had a close family friend who was a physician so Randy suggested I let him in on the recent news. He was helpful in answering a few questions and offered to arrange an appointment with a surgeon in his medical complex. I was grateful he could get me in early the following week and I was instructed to pick up my mammogram and ultrasound films and a copy of the report. I could expedite this process by hand carrying the information to my appointment. Taking care of this quickly was critical. I wanted to have my biopsy done before our trip to Utah. I was anxious to have all of this behind me so I could enjoy the rest of the summer. Besides my family and physician friend, I chose not to tell anyone else. Why concern others before I knew the outcome? I was still very hopeful and confident that all would be fine.

On Sunday, I felt prompted to call another good friend and doctor who had performed my hysterectomy several years before. I chided myself for not thinking of him sooner. He was well known and respected in the medical community and would have a good recommendation for a surgeon. Most importantly, I wouldn't hesitate to follow his advice.

Dr. Burton was extremely helpful and gave me the name of a surgeon he highly recommended. I told him of my other appointment with a surgeon early next week and he advised that I go with an open mind and see how I felt. He said there were many good surgeons, but it was important to feel confident in my choice. He continued to assure me that it wasn't uncommon, and actually quite important to shop around when it came to making decisions concerning one's health. I was grateful for his advice and compassion for my situation and I told him I'd keep him informed.

Confiding in these two friends helped me not feel so lost and alone as I took the necessary steps to accomplish my goal of having my breast biopsied as soon as possible. I was quite certain it was benign and the sooner I could prove that and get on with my life, the better.

At times like this, optimism is a good companion.

After what seemed like a very long weekend, I awoke Monday morning ready to tackle the day. I called the imaging lab to arrange a time to pick up my reports and films. I received a call from my friend informing me I had an appointment with a surgeon on Tuesday morning. I thought that everything was falling into place beautifully and by the end of the week I should have the results of the biopsy and this nightmare behind me. Only later did I learn that an imaging lab would perform the biopsy and not a surgeon. Since the day the radiologist had first given me her report, I felt like I was running in circles, trying to find a logical direction to take, and I was confused with the whole process. Was it because I didn't ask enough questions? It's hard to know what kind of questions to ask when you are entering a world that is foreign and everyone assumes you know what to do. Maybe my mind was so muddled that I wasn't catching the clues I needed to proceed.

When it was time, I drove to the lab, anxious to pick up my reports and films. Even though I called ahead, I still had to wait for everything to be gathered. Did they have any idea how much I hate to wait? Finally, they were in my possession and I hurried out to the car. I really hadn't thought ahead to what I was going to do once I had them. Should I open the large brown envelope and read the report? Would I even be able to understand it?

June in Arizona is hot, but I was so anxious to view the contents of the envelope that I decided to read it before leaving the parking lot for my next errand. I gently peeled up the metal clasps that secured the flap, allowing me access to the classified information inside. Ever so carefully, I removed the two pages of details that summarized the hour I spent sharing images of my breast. I was vaguely aware of my stuffy environment as I scanned the ultrasound report. Reading the first few paragraphs, most of which I didn't understand, provided a measure of hope. So far, nothing seemed unusual. However, when I turned to the next page, I felt like I was being slapped in the face as I read the phrases: "highly suggestive of malignancy", "highly recommend an MRI prior to surgical planning" and "evaluate not only extent of disease but also allow for screening of the right breast for cancer". Hastily I stuffed the report back in the brown manila envelope and threw it on the seat beside me as if it were poisonous. I tried to shake the words from my mind. I started the car and left quickly, wanting to get as far away as possible from the imaging center, but I could not get away from what I'd just read.

Wanting to clear the mounting panic in my head, I drove to a nearby convenience store and parked. I had originally intended to pick up a few things on my way home from securing the report, and was attempting to resume my plans like nothing was amiss. I went in and walked aimlessly around, trying to collect my thoughts. I jumped when my cell phone rang. It was Randy calling to see how I was doing.

"Hi. Just checking in on how your day is going. Did you get the report?"

As usual, his caring voice brought a sense of clarity to the situation. I tried to ground myself, but couldn't hold back the tears as I shared with him words from the report.

"I did get the report, and I couldn't help but try to read it. It doesn't sound good, Randy. I don't know what all the terms mean, but I do understand the words 'malignant' and 'surgical planning', and worst of all, 'cancer'. I need you to look at it and tell me what all this means."

"I will, sweetheart. As soon as I get home, we'll go over it together. Don't jump to conclusions. It usually sounds worse than it is."

I knew with Randy's medical background as a dentist, he would be able to decipher some of the terminology. I could hope that when he read the report, those words would suddenly be gone, or wouldn't mean what they appeared to mean. I tried to remain positive, but when it was in black and white print, it was hard to maintain my desire to be optimistic. I still had to hope that the biopsy would prove the lump to be benign and this bad dream would soon pass. Unable to concentrate or hold back my tears, I got out of the store and drove home.

The day seemed long as I lost my resolve to accomplish any of the things that needed to be done. I didn't want to alarm my children about this discovery so I went to lunch with one of my good friends, Lauri. I decided to share my concerns with her as I knew she would understand, having lost her husband to cancer a few years ago. It seemed to ease the burden to divulge my fears to a friend. Even though the news was a surprise, Lauri was an empathetic listener and provided some encouraging insights. She reminded me that if I did have breast cancer, modern research provided very positive outcomes.

Since it would still be several hours before Randy got home, I drove over to Monica's house, hoping she would be there. Monica and I had been close friends for years and I could tell her anything. Being a nurse, I was confident she would be able to understand more of the medical terms and explain them. As we sat outside on her wicker porch furniture, I watched her face as she scanned the report. When she finished reading, Monica looked at me with a pained look and softly said, "Claudia, the report is suggesting a strong possibility of breast cancer. You need to have your breast biopsied as soon as possible."

It wasn't what I wanted to hear but I needed to start facing the possibility of what might be ahead. Sharing the news with two of my best friends gave me added strength as Randy and I sat together that evening to discuss the probability of cancer as indicated by the report. It grieved my soul to see my dear husband valiantly remaining strong for me when I knew the dreadful fear he must be experiencing as well. With the words, *malignant*, *surgery*, and *cancer* weighing heavily on my mind, I found it hard to sleep. That little cancer demon kept making a racket, tormenting me with its teasing.

The next morning couldn't come fast enough. I was consumed with an intense desire to get everything figured out as soon as possible. I think it was the first time in my life I didn't feel in control and it was driving me crazy. As I drove to the surgeon's office, I prayed for guidance to know if this was the direction I should take. I chided myself for feeling rushed. Instinctively I knew I should calm down and take whatever time I needed to make an educated decision. My logical self was not winning however, and my mind swirled with the uncertainty of the situation and my impatience in proving I was not facing cancer.

The office smelled new and was clean and neat. I filled out the necessary paper work and gave the receptionist all the information I had brought. I was alone in the waiting room and didn't expect it to be long before I saw the doctor. As I waited, I envisioned him pouring over the report and disc containing the scans, preparing to give me his recommendation. I was finally shown into the exam room and again I waited. In the distance, I could hear construction workers using electrical tools and grimaced at the irony of such background noise in a surgeon's office.

Finally, a nurse entered, instructing me to undress from the waist up, handing me a thin paper gown. As I sat on the hard table, I desperately tried to keep my thoughts positive. I felt uncomfortable meeting a new doctor, but quickly realized I better get accustomed to it. When he finally entered, I looked at him circumspectly to get a feel for the situation. After quickly introducing himself, he sat down and read the report I had brought, dashing my theory that he had been preparing during my long wait. I knew he was through reading when he grunted and asked me to lie down on the exam table. Without much effort, he found a lump on my left breast. I had never felt it before so he directed my hand to the exact location.

"That is quite a large lump and I'm surprised you didn't notice it sooner. It should have been detected on a mammogram even a year ago," he stated accusingly.

Since first discovering I needed a biopsy, I had blamed myself for my condition. Why didn't I pay more attention to my body, and why did I wait so long to address the changes in my breast when I finally took time to notice? I didn't need this doctor to make me feel guilty. I had already accomplished that on my own and was not impressed with his callous approach.

In a very business-like tone, the surgeon quickly went over several different procedures and options, but I found myself unable to follow or retain the information. He spoke rapidly using terms I've never heard.

After I dressed and walked out of the exam room, I saw him in the hall and expressed my desire to have a biopsy as soon as possible. He directed me to his nurse who remarked she would get around to scheduling it later that afternoon due to an overload of morning paperwork. Not easily giving up, I explained again how important it was to address this problem immediately. She shrugged and said she would be contacting me. When she did get around to calling me to schedule a biopsy more than a week later, I had already moved on.

As I look back on this scene, I'm sure I was as frustrating to them as they were to me. They see patients all day long that have needs. It is unfortunate that some physicians lose sight of the fact their patients are human beings to whom all this is new and frightening. A little genuine compassion and kindness between physician and patient goes a long way.

I left that office feeling I had wasted a lot of time, except for being able to scratch this doctor's name off the list. It is also clear, looking back, that the surgeon's attitude had rubbed off on the staff.

When I got home I called Amber, the nurse practitioner that had referred me for a diagnostic mammogram in the first place. She had received the report from the imaging center and immediately took my call. My timing was right for once as I wasn't put on hold or asked to leave a message. She expressed her concern that I get a biopsy as soon as possible and said she would make the necessary calls and rush the process.

Having her undivided attention for a moment, I asked, "Amber, how could this happen when I was always faithful about getting my yearly check-ups?"

Her answer didn't make me feel any better. "There are a lot of fast growing cancers out there. It can happen to anyone. While I make the arrangements for a biopsy, you need to call and make an appointment right away with a surgeon to discuss the results as soon as they're available."

"Do you have any recommendations for a good surgeon?" I asked hopefully.

Without hesitation she responded, "We highly recommend Dr. Deyden. You can't go wrong with him."

I felt a surge of hope as everything started fitting together. Dr. Deyden was the same surgeon Dr. Burton had endorsed. I was beginning to sense some degree of peace for the first time, knowing that Amber was arranging the biopsy and I had the name of a competent surgeon. Just being recommended by others I trusted gave me the confidence to call his office and make an appointment, settling one more worry.

It was Tuesday, June 30. We were planning to leave for Utah on July 3. When I received a call later that day from the imaging center to schedule the biopsy, I found the earliest I could get in was Monday, July 6. This meant we would have to delay our trip for a few days. If not, I would have to wait and wonder the duration of the vacation.

Randy said to go ahead and make the appointment for July 6 as early in the morning as I could, and we would drive to Utah after the biopsy was completed. I got an appointment at 7:00 a.m. and since the only instructions after a biopsy were to rest and apply ice packs, I knew that could be easily accomplished in a car on the way to see my children and grandchildren.

I was also able to make an appointment with the surgeon when Randy was free to accompany me a few days after we returned from vacation. For the first time since my mammogram on the previous Friday, I finally felt some degree of calmness knowing I had done everything I could do up to this point. I decided to let the matter rest and focus on preparing for our trip and making plans for the fourth of July since we would now be in town. I also concentrated on having positive thoughts and not allowing myself to worry about something I couldn't control. This was a whole lot easier to decide than to do, but with the biopsy arranged and the surgeon chosen and scheduled, my state of mind greatly improved.

On the fourth of July, we ended up attending an early morning breakfast and program sponsored by our church. In attendance was an elderly man that had recently been diagnosed with cancer. His hair was already thinning and he looked lean and pale. I shuddered with the possibility that I could be in his position in a few months. I was impressed with his high spirits despite all he had already endured. This gentleman was still coming to social functions, and maintaining his jolly, friendly personality. He had no idea how carefully I was observing his positive attitude.

Monday morning, July 6, came quickly with all the packing and arrangements that take place when going out of town. Early in the morning Randy drove me to the biopsy appointment. It was similar to the place where I had my mammogram, but was decorated with women in mind. The gown I was given to wear was not the typical crinkly paper kind but was made of light cotton material, scattered with pink rosebuds. For some reason, being draped in soft cloth instead of paper brought a sense of comfort to the situation.

I didn't know what to expect when it came to a biopsy. I was anxious to have it done and over, and one step closer to alleviating my worries. The results of this test would be the deciding factor that determined my fate. If it turned out benign, I could continue on with my life as I knew it and never look back. But if. . . . I wouldn't allow myself to think past "if". I was still trying to ignore the little cancer demon in my mind, but it seemed to be amused at my distress and was refusing to leave.

I was directed to a room and asked to lie on a table with my left arm over my head. A pleasant, elderly woman came in and introduced herself as a doctor. She radiated an aura of calmness and I felt safe in her care. As we visited, I explained that all this had occurred since my last yearly check-up. I wanted people to know I hadn't been slothful in taking care of myself, still holding on to the guilt I felt. She assured me she saw many cases where cancer appeared between yearly mammograms. I was comforted knowing I hadn't done anything wrong and wasn't to blame for where I was that morning.

She explained the procedure and the importance of holding still, and then administered a shot of Lidocaine to deaden the area. After the shot, she excused herself, promising to return in about fifteen minutes, after the Lidocaine had time to do its job. A nurse stayed with me and chatted casually to keep me company, a kindness for which I was grateful.

When the doctor returned, she started the biopsy, her work guided by an ultrasound machine. I closed my eyes during the entire procedure. I didn't want to see the needle or any of the other instruments she was about to use. Hearing the instruments being freed from their sterilized packages was enough to feed my imagination. It's a good thing I had no idea at the time that this was just the beginning of my affair with needles. All I felt was pressure and the entire process was completed in a matter of minutes. The nurse instructed me in the proper care of the biopsied area, and we were on our way. To say I was relieved to finally have this appointment behind me was a flagrant understatement. My mind would not rest however, until I learned the verdict.

The trip to Utah was uneventful and I didn't experience much discomfort from the early morning appointment. It was helpful to apply ice packs and I was grateful for the chance to rest. I smiled as I remembered the instructions the nurse rehearsed in front of Randy. I wasn't to lift anything and basically rest all day. No housework, no preparing dinner, etc. I was a queen for the day. Since Randy always treated me like a queen, I didn't have to worry about the directions being followed.

That night as we arrived at our daughter's home in Utah, the excitement of seeing my family overshadowed any nagging worries I had about my impending prognosis. I was excited for this time our family had to be together and I was determined it would be a memorable reunion. It had been a long drive and I was grateful to finally get the chance to go to bed and rest.

Some days of our lives are ordinary, while others have significant meaning. This year, July 7, 2009 proved to be both meaningful and memorable, a day I will never forget. First of all, it was my husband's birthday. When I asked him several days earlier what he wanted for his birthday, he said, "For you to be well." I hoped I could accommodate his sweet request. July 7, 2009 will also be remembered for being the day I received the call.

We awoke early and had breakfast with our daughter, Autumn, and her family. Our oldest daughter, Julie, had followed us in her van from Arizona with her five little ones. Her husband was unable to make the trip due to his work schedule at the hospital. My second daughter, Kimberly, also stayed behind in Arizona due to work responsibilities. We enjoyed our visit as we waited for our other children who lived in the area to arrive. Doug and Whitney joined us soon for a short visit, but had to leave for work. We planned to get together with them later that evening. When my daughter Kristy and her little boy Justus arrived, we all decided to go to a nearby park and have a picnic. The weather was wonderful and it would be great to be outside with my family. To keep things easy, we purchased fried chicken and sides at a local fast food restaurant on our way to the park. With our large group, I was grateful for the outdoor picnic tables that easily accommodated everyone, as well as all the spills.

When we finished eating and cleaning up, the children eagerly headed for the playground equipment while the rest of us threw down blankets on the soft grass. Randy chose a spot under the shade of a nearby tree while the women stayed closer to the playground to keep an eye on the little ones. As I plopped my purse down on a bench, it occurred to me that I should check the ringer volume on my cell phone. I wasn't really expecting to hear the results of my biopsy so soon, but just in case, I didn't want to miss the call.

I took out my camera and photographed my grandchildren as they played together, happy to be outside on such a beautiful day. There was a slight breeze and it was at least twenty degrees cooler than the oppressive heat of Arizona. I loved visiting with my children and immersed myself in the joy I felt being together in such peaceful surroundings, far away from the frightful events of the past two weeks.

The magic of the occasion was abruptly shattered when I heard my cell phone ring. It startled me and I ran to grab it out of my purse. I didn't recognize the number, but the call was from Arizona and I felt a pit in my stomach. Cautiously answering and hearing my nurse practitioner's voice, I walked to a nearby tree, away from the others so I could hear clearly. I was desperately trying to quiet the rising panic in my mind while striving to grasp every word and read the tone in her voice, wondering if early news was good or bad.

"Hi. This is Amber. I'm sorry I have to call you. I wish I could meet with you in person."

So far, the conversation was not starting out well. "That's fine," I assured her trying to keep my voice steady. "You didn't have much choice since I'm on vacation."

Amber continued, "I just received the results of your breast biopsy this morning and the tumor is cancerous."

There it was. Simple, short…. Cancer.

With one word, all my hope was shattered into tiny pieces and my chest felt like someone had slammed it with a brick. My surroundings turned from bright greens and blues to dull grays.

I suddenly realized she was waiting for me to respond. "OK. Where do I go from here?"

"It is very important to see a surgeon as soon as you get home from your trip. Have you chosen one yet?"

"I used your recommendation and have an appointment with Dr. Deyden."

"Good. Until then, there is nothing more you can do. Just enjoy the time with your family and try not to worry."

She shared some details about the type of cancer I had, but my mind didn't comprehend or remember a word she said. I was trying desperately to think of questions to ask, but since I hadn't expected the call to go this direction, my mind was blank.

"I'm so sorry I had to call you with this news," she tenderly apologized again.

"That's okay. I really appreciate all you've done for me." I could tell this was not a call she looked forward to making, and I tried to relieve her uneasiness, despite my pain.

"Let me know if you have any questions. You can contact me anytime."

With that, we both hung up. I stared at the gnarled roots that protruded above the ground next to the old tree I was near. I felt like kicking them. I wanted to scream to clear my head of the words I just heard. In the background, I could hear my family laughing and talking, oblivious to the life changing phone call I had just received. What do you do when you just learn you have cancer? What do you tell your loved ones and how? I was never more grateful that I was not alone.

As I walked back to the group I noticed that Kristy's husband, James, had arrived, so I welcomed him with a hug and simply said to those in hearing distance, "I just found out I have cancer."

The words hung in the air, heavy and solemn. The next thing I knew, I was embraced by my grown children. Tears did not fall immediately as each one tried to assimilate the actual meaning of what I just said. The silence was piercing as we embraced in stunned unbelief. I'm sure their minds were filled with many thoughts, but none were expressed at that time. What do you say to your mom who has just found out she has cancer?

In the distance, I saw my husband still resting under a tree. Today was his birthday and grief engulfed me as I realized I was unable to give him the one present he wanted. Should I wait until tomorrow to tell him? That was an impossible choice now as I had already hastily told the others. It occurred to me that I should have told him first. If I had thought of that, I could have waited for a better day to let everyone know, but my need to not be alone in my anguish kept me from thinking things through. My mind did find relief however in not having to deal with this by myself, even for a day, and I was grateful for the love and support of my family from the very beginning.

As I walked over to Randy, I silently prayed that he would be comforted as he heard the results of my biopsy. I joined him on the soft blanket and searched my mind for just the right way to start. I decided it was best to be direct.

"Hi," I began, tenderly taking his hand in mine. "I just got a call from Amber. She received the results of my biopsy and--" I paused, not sure if I could choke out the necessary words, "I do have cancer."

Randy softly squeezed my hand, and then took me in his arms. I buried my head in his chest, never wanting to leave the strength of his embrace. I was overcome with sorrow, wishing someone would wake me from this nightmare. For the moment, in the protective arms of my sweetheart, I allowed myself to grieve, letting the tears fall freely. It was one of the few times I permitted myself to do that.

When my tears finally slowed, we sat for a while in silence. Words were not necessary as we connected heart to heart. I knew beyond a doubt that, with his love and support, I could find the strength to face the enemy that invaded my body. I would never be alone in this fight. I realized this was a priceless blessing and in my grief and turmoil I was nevertheless profoundly grateful for such a wonderful husband.

I remember silently watching the puffy clouds form different shapes above us. How rarely I took the time to slow down and notice nature and I was grateful for how calm the clouds made me feel. It was a time of fortification as I soaked in the strength provided by my husband's embrace. Finally, he gently kissed me and whispered, "You are going to be just fine." He said it with such conviction that I believed him. I had to believe.

Since all my immediate family wasn't present that day at the park, I needed to pull myself together and let the others know. My daughter Kimberly would not take the news well and I didn't look forward to telling her over the phone. As a child, she worried about me whenever I was out of her sight. She was especially sensitive to illness and pain and I wanted to be there to help her through the shock of my diagnosis. Waiting to tell her in person, however, was not an option. She would want to know along with the others. My call to her was difficult as I tried to sound cheerful and positive.

That evening I had a chance to tell Doug and Whitney that I was facing cancer. As I shared the results of my biopsy, I assured them all would be well. I tried to be optimistic knowing that my only son would take the news especially hard. Doug has always been protective of me and the worry showed in his face. I found myself going overboard to convince him all would be fine. By the end of the day, I was worn out trying to portray an overly positive attitude in front of my family. The truth was, my future was uncertain and I was scared.

*July 14, 2009*

*Dear Journal,*

*I met Dr. Deyden today. He carefully and scientifically explained why we should remove both breasts. If I want to rid my body of cancer and have the best chance of surviving, I have to eliminate the source. The only way to effectively accomplish this is with a double mastectomy.*

*I totally trust his judgment and while my mind completely agrees with all his reasoning, my heart is light years behind.*

2

# COPING

The remainder of our vacation in Utah was filled with wonderful moments and memories. We didn't talk about my newly diagnosed cancer, but tried to go forward as if nothing were amiss. We all put on our happy faces and made the most of each day. I knew my children would worry less if I was optimistic and cheerful. I was the one setting the tone and I wanted our time together to be like past vacations.

I didn't want the trip to end. I knew that I would be going home to doctor appointments, decisions, and surgery. I would also have to tell the principal of the school where I taught about my diagnosis. I planned to keep on teaching, but I would need a substitute to begin the year while I recovered from surgery. Then there was the possibility of chemotherapy. I didn't know yet if treatments would be required or how often. Those were answers not even the doctors could give until after surgery and the extent of the cancer had been determined. I tried not to think about the road ahead, but my mind would often tip toe down unpaved paths during quiet moments. I knew I needed to concentrate on the present. Too soon this diversion would end.

I found that during the daytime hours when I was surrounded by my family, I rarely thought about my cancer diagnosis. Each time its dark tentacles tried to capture my attention, I pushed them away with family involvement. At night, I readily welcomed sleep so I wouldn't have to think about cancer, and most nights I was so exhausted from the day's activities that sleep came easily. The wee hours of the morning were the worst as I typically awoke before anyone else. Those early hours allowed too much time to think and ponder my situation, causing a murky gloom to descend upon me.

One such morning I took my cell phone and left the basement where we were staying. I sat outside beneath the beautiful Wasatch Mountains in Provo, Utah with the sun barely rising over the tops. It was July and I found it intriguing to still see patches of snow on the tip of the highest peaks. There was something calming about a brand-new day when most of the world was sleeping, except for the birds that filled the air with song and activity.

I watched two little sparrows playfully flitting back and forth just a few feet away from where I sat. How cheerful they were. As they teased each other, I longingly wished I could feel so carefree. The burden of my diagnosis was wearing on me, and I coveted their lighthearted existence.

As I sat there, I decided to call Cindy, a long-time friend. We were inseparable when we lived as neighbors in Colorado, and our friendship never wavered, even though she now lived in Virginia and my home was clear across the country in Arizona. She had been diagnosed with cancer nearly three years ago and had endured many dark months of chemotherapy and its side effects. I felt the need to talk to someone who had been where I now stood. Since she lived in a different time zone, it wouldn't be too early to call.

Searching for her name on my cell phone, I held my breath wondering how to start this conversation. When I heard her cheerful voice on the other end, I immediately knew my talk with her would be just what I needed.

"Cindy, it's so good to hear your voice! You have no idea how much I need to talk to you."

"It's great to talk to you too! It's been awhile. What's going on?"

"Right now I'm in Provo with most of the family. We're having a great time together, but that's not why I called." I hesitated, fumbling for the best way to tell her. Knowing Cindy, being direct would be best.

"I just found out earlier this week that I have breast cancer," I blurted.

There are no words that adequately describe the depth of sorrow in her voice, the voice of someone who had traveled the road I was now beginning.

"Oh Claudia. I'm so sorry."

Cindy and I spent more than an hour on the phone, sharing feelings that only friends walking the same path can understand. Before ending our conversation that day, Cindy offered two pieces of advice that proved to be invaluable as I prepared to begin my journey with cancer.

"Now Claudia, don't slip into the 'Why me?' syndrome. Getting cancer is not a result of anything you did. Don't expend energy on feeling sorry for yourself," she wisely counseled.

"Next, keep a notebook by your bed. Jot down any questions you have so you don't forget to discuss them with your doctor. Be sure to keep track of any adverse side-effects you experience. Many times, reactions to drugs you are given can be alleviated by letting the medical team know. You don't have to suffer in silence."

"I can't tell you how sharing this burden with you has helped me. Little did we know during our carefree days in Colorado that we'd both battle cancer. Will you do one thing for me?" I pleaded.

"I will do anything for you," she assured me.

"Pray for me to have the strength to endure whatever is in my future."

"I will. You know I will."

Cindy turned out to be my anchor as well as my comic relief during the following year. If I ever began to feel sorry for myself, she had the uncanny talent of grounding me and helping me find the humor in any situation. I found myself texting her many times during my treatments, knowing I could say whatever I wanted and she would understand. She sent numerous light-hearted cards that lifted my spirits and made me laugh. I think God places people in our lives that double as angels when we need them most.

Our vacation in Utah came to an end far too quickly, as all vacations do. I reluctantly said good-bye to the family I wouldn't be seeing anytime soon. Leaving was more difficult than in times past for all of us. I knew I had their support, but necessity dictated it could only be from a distance. Each mile we drove south towards Arizona placed me closer to reality and the future I dreaded.

Upon arriving back home in Mesa, I did all the things people usually do when returning from a trip. I had endless piles of laundry and cleaning to keep me busy, not to mention grocery shopping and restocking the fridge. These mundane tasks helped pass the slow as molasses days before my first visit with the surgeon.

Three days after arriving home, Randy and I were finally sitting in the surgeon's office where I hoped to find answers to my many questions. When Dr. Deyden walked in, I immediately felt comfortable with him although he wasn't at all what I had pictured. He was small in stature, probably no taller than five feet, eight inches, and looked to be in his mid-sixties. Dr. Deyden flashed that teasing smile I soon grew to love and said that he had received a call from Dr. Burton. He was given strict instructions to take good care of me. I could tell he would anyway, but was pleased to know my friend had called ahead.

After examining me and checking the records that had been sent to him, he spoke to us in great detail about the kind of breast cancer I had and his surgical recommendations. He drew diagrams for us, explaining the reasons he felt a total mastectomy of the affected breast was the only choice and that he wouldn't be able to save the nipple due to the location of the cancer. I learned I had lobular breast cancer, less common than ductal, which was difficult to detect on a mammogram, especially with the density of my breasts. He assured me he had seen other cases where breast cancer appeared after a yearly check-up and could surface as early as three months following imaging. What a difference Dr. Deyden was from the first surgeon I saw. Instead of placing responsibility for having cancer on my shoulders, Dr. Deyden made sure I knew it wasn't my fault.

After studying the hastily drawn diagrams and listening intently, I asked him if surgery would be followed by chemo. He was frank when he told me I would most definitely receive four to six sessions of chemotherapy, depending on the number of lymph nodes involved, which would be determined at the time of surgery. He explained how they would test the primary lymph node for cancer during surgery and if it was cancerous, all the lymph nodes under my left arm would be removed. They would be sent to pathology to determine the total number affected.

Next I asked probably the most pressing question on my mind. "Will I lose my hair?"

"Yes, but it'll grow back," he remarked as casually as if we were talking about newly mown grass.

Trying to suppress the panic mounting in my mind from the uncomfortable but undeniable fact that my hair would be falling out, I quickly diverted the conversation back to the upcoming surgery. Strange, but I think I was more concerned about losing my hair, which would grow back, than my breasts, which wouldn't.

After patiently answering all the questions Randy and I could think of, Dr. Deyden led us to the front to schedule surgery. I was surprised he could fit me in the very next week on a Wednesday at 3:00 p.m. He also ordered an MRI of the right breast to detect possible signs of cancer. He explained that in many cases when cancer is found in one breast it is already beginning in the other, or will soon follow. He proposed we be pro-active and have both breasts removed to eliminate trouble down the road. I didn't want to go through this twice, so we agreed to his recommendation. We left Dr. Deyden's office with the decision to have a bilateral mastectomy.

Neither Randy nor I said much on the ride home from the surgeon's office. There was so much to digest and think about and we were both lost in our thoughts. To me, the whole thing was surreal. I couldn't believe this was really happening. Going through chemo was something I read or heard about, but never imagined being a part of my life. I couldn't envision being bald and how would I handle such a drastic change in my appearance? What would it be like to be completely flat? I was never well endowed, but I did like my nicely shaped breasts. I was aware of reconstructive surgery, but that was an avenue that hadn't been discussed yet. Since all of this was hard for me to process, I simply became matter-of-fact when explaining to others the outcome of our visit with the surgeon. It was as if I had stepped out of my body and was an observer without emotion.

A few days after my appointment with Dr. Deyden, I had a conversation about my diagnosis and surgical plans with Dr. Dinsdale, our family physician. Being a friend as well as my doctor for several years, he voiced compassion and concern. Giving one last piece of advice as he was leaving our home, he said, "Claudia, remember, it is what it is."

That's true, I thought, but I wasn't ready to accept that and wished like heck it wasn't what it was. Those words stung, yet I couldn't deny their reality.

With surgery around the corner, I knew I couldn't waste time getting things ready for the upcoming school year. Surgery was scheduled for July 22 and teachers were to report the first week of August. School began the second week of August. After surgery, I would need six weeks to recover so it was apparent I wouldn't be present for the first few weeks of school, the most important days in setting the tone for the entire year. There was always a great deal to be done in preparation for the start of a new year, and organizing for a substitute added more to my already full plate. Time was ticking and it was imperative I let the principal know of my situation and solicit her much needed support. I also decided to confide in my good friend and colleague, Peggy. Guessing she was working at the school already, I drove over.

As soon as she heard of my cancer diagnosis, Peggy offered to help set up my classroom and get things ready for the first few weeks. Peggy's willingness to lighten my load was a true sacrifice for she had her own classroom to prepare and lessons to plan. Relieving some of the weight of the impending school year was truly a gift, but no one could take away the burden of telling my principal. Sue had to know, and this talk would not be easy.

After rehearsing in my head what I would say, I finally mustered the courage to walk to the principal's office to see if she was available. Was I sweating because I was nervous, or was it the stifling, hot July day? Half hoping she wasn't in, I knocked lightly on her door. Sue answered with a huge smile on her face, genuinely happy to see me. It didn't take long to feel at ease in her presence as she casually chatted about the upcoming year.

I had a great deal of respect for this woman and I loved working for her. Sue genuinely cared about the adults and children under her supervision. How I hated to spoil her cheerful mood with my burdens, and the possible ramifications for the upcoming school year. When it was my turn to contribute to the conversation, I lost courage and took a detour, stalling for more time.

"So, tell me about your summer, Sue. Did you get a chance to get away?"

"No. I was planning to go to Colorado for a week, but I ended up staying here to conduct interviews for a fourth-grade position. The work load never ends. How about you?"

The question didn't allow for further delays, so I decided to press forward with the reason for my visit.

"Well, we went to Utah to see family. Before going I took care of my yearly female check-up and discovered--." Again, that uncomfortable pause. Will this ever get easy to say? "Ummm, well, I found out I have breast cancer."

I paused to let it sink in. The look on her face was a combination of disbelief and sorrow. She was speechless, so I continued.

"The prognosis is good since they caught it early." I found myself repeating this statement often, even though I didn't really know how early it had been caught or if it had already invaded other areas of my body. This was my way of attempting to be positive and relieve the shock for those finding out for the first time.

Before she had a chance to respond to that statement, I quickly continued. "I will be having a bilateral mastectomy on July 22nd so I'll have to miss the first few weeks of school. After that, I'm not sure what I'll be facing, but I can assure you I won't miss any more school than necessary. I plan to carry on and make this year work. I won't let you down, or my class of second-graders."

Sue was visibly shaken by the unexpected news and it took her a few minutes to respond. How I disliked putting people in this position. If it were possible, I'd face this trial without anyone knowing, but cancer is a difficult disease to hide.

After composing herself, Sue assured me that I didn't need to worry. She would be there to offer any assistance. I knew Sue would understand, but I was also aware she took pride in the school being one of the best in the district. She expected outstanding performances from the teachers she carefully selected and hired. The last thing I wanted was for her to doubt my ability to achieve her expectations, and I was sensitive to the possibility of causing disappointment to anyone, including myself.

Walking out of the office that day, I rejoiced in crossing another hurdle in my attempt to put things in order before surgery. I felt like the track athlete who had successfully jumped several hurdles, with endless hurdles to clear, stretching far into the horizon. I was already so very tired.

After sharing the news with Sue, I went to my classroom to begin the process of creating bulletin boards and arranging the room for the beginning of the school year. I had to start from scratch as the custodians used the summer to wax the tile and clean the carpet. All the desks and chairs were stacked against the wall. Before I knew it, Peggy showed up with Lori, another good friend. I had known Lori for years and called upon her to substitute the few times I needed to be absent. She had graduated in education but chose the freedom of taking substitute jobs when she was needed. Lori and I were similar in our temperaments and philosophy of education and she was familiar with how I ran my classroom. Without wasting words, she saw I needed help and pitched in immediately to assist with the mammoth task of transforming my room.

While working together, Lori casually mentioned her desire to become more involved in school this year. Her oldest daughter was now married and her second daughter was away at college. She had more time on her hands and wished to come and help in my classroom, especially with the challenges I would be facing. I suddenly felt I was talking to the person that would answer my need for a constant, dependable substitute. I asked about her availability and if she would be interested in helping me out. I knew it would be better for the children to have the same substitute when I was gone, and it would be much easier to work with someone who knew my style of teaching and could pick up the slack if necessary. Lori was excited for the opportunity and I knew it wasn't a coincidence she walked in that day. I probably should give Peggy some credit for that as well.

Having found a consistent, reliable substitute gave me renewed energy with the extra weight off my shoulders. I could begin right away to prepare lessons for the beginning of the year and have time to explain them as well as classroom procedures. Despite the magnitude of the recent news things were beginning to fall into place. We continued working side by side that day, accomplishing my huge list together.

News spreads fast and it wasn't long before the school community learned I had breast cancer. I have lived in this neighborhood for seventeen years. My children attended school and church activities here and we are acquainted with many of the families. I was overwhelmed with the countless offers to help, not only in preparing for the school year, but getting through what loomed ahead.

During one of the trips to prepare my room, I noticed several mothers and their older children cleaning out the school garden that Peggy and I coordinate for our first and second-grade students each year. At the end of summer, the neglected plot of ground was overrun with weeds and dried up plants left over from the previous spring garden. In the past, Peggy and I tackled the job of weeding and clearing out the mess, which was no minor undertaking. This year I couldn't help her. The garden was an eyesore in its present condition and had to be taken care of before the start of school. It was a supreme act of service to have the garden cleaned and ready to plant again in just a matter of an hour with all the volunteer help. As I watched others accomplish what I could not, I was filled with gratitude to be the recipient of so much love and service. My mind filled with the words from a favorite hymn, "Oh to grace, how great the debtor, daily I'm constrained to be."

Besides trying to prepare for a new school year, I had the additional challenge of fitting in required pre-surgery tests and appointments. The first on my list was the MRI on my right, unaffected breast, ordered by Dr. Deyden. I didn't know what to expect and little did I realize this would be the first of many imaging experiences. I was a reluctant stranger to this new world of appointments and tests, followed by the often-lengthy wait for results. I was definitely not a fan.

Entering the room on the day of my MRI, I was amazed at the massive machine. The technician was prepared for me, having arranged the table to accommodate my right breast as I lay on my stomach. Once in place, I was told to turn my head to the left and put my right arm up over my head. As he placed pillows to support my left arm I could tell he was trying to make me as comfortable as possible. After all, I had to lie perfectly still for about twenty minutes.

Achieving the correct position on the hard table, we were ready to begin. As the table slid under the huge tube, I closed my eyes to prevent claustrophobia. I reasoned that if I didn't know how enclosed I was, I wouldn't care. I tried to be completely cooperative and not move at all, but I found myself becoming overly aware of my breathing. After all, breathing does require movement of the chest and it's hard to "breathe normally" when you're worried you might be moving too much with each breath. This awareness made it difficult to relax. In addition, I experienced the overwhelming urge to open my eyes. It took lots of determination not to do so. I was afraid how I might react to my constricted surroundings.

Within a minute after entering the tube, I began hearing the strangest noises. They were random and different in tones and length. It began with sharp staccato tapings, then pounding, followed by rapid clicking noises and then a welcomed silence. Without warning, the noises would begin again, causing me to jump. I had heard of patients having to repeat the entire procedure due to moving too much. The very thought of having to endure this again caused me to augment my resolve to hold perfectly still.

When the MRI was complete, I was assisted in returning to an upright position. No mention was made of repeating the test, so I presumed I held still enough despite everything. I detected a certain look in the technician's eyes as he excused me to get dressed and I speculated I would be hearing some not so pleasant news soon. I don't know why, but I was beginning to think I could guess results by studying how the nurse or technician looked at me and how they spoke when it was time to leave. I was probably just imagining it, but I would soon know if my hunch was right.

My youngest daughter, Brittany, was preparing for her senior year of high school with much more excitement than I was preparing for my upcoming surgery. She was my only child left at home and we had both been looking forward to another year of shopping trips, eating out, and long talks before she left home for college. I was determined to keep things as normal as possible so we planned our back to school shopping trip for clothes, like we do every summer. I didn't have many extra days before I relinquished control of my life, but I wanted to make the most of the time we had together.

It was the Friday before my surgery and we were shopping in a typical store that catered to teenagers. As soon as you walk in, loud music prohibits any communication or clear thinking, so I was surprised that I even heard my cell phone ring. I excused myself to go outside so I could hear the voice addressing me, only to find it was the nurse from my surgeon's office. She informed me that something was found on my right breast during the MRI and I would need to have the mass biopsied. The earliest they could schedule it was for next Tuesday, the day before my scheduled surgery.

I couldn't understand the purpose of going through another biopsy when we had already decided to remove both breasts. I expressed my opinion to the nurse and she must have told Dr. Deyden because as soon as I had joined Brittany in the store, my phone rang again. Not often does a patient talk to a doctor over the phone directly, so I was surprised to hear his voice. Since he is soft spoken with a slight accent, I immediately exited the noisy environment and stepped outside. As I did so, an airplane chose that moment to fly directly overhead, making it impossible to hear what he said. Embarrassed, I asked him to repeat himself.

"Claudia, I remember we talked about going ahead and removing the right breast at the same time we remove the left. If you want, we can skip the biopsy and go ahead with the surgery as planned."

Sensing he was not completely comfortable with that I inquired, "What do you think I should do?"

"Well, to be honest, I would prefer getting the right breast biopsied. If you don't and the pathology report deems the mass to be malignant. I will have to go back in and check the right lymph nodes for cancer. It would involve additional surgery."

"I don't want to do that. Let's go ahead and get the biopsy."

"You know this means we'll have to reschedule your surgery. We won't have the results of the biopsy until the end of the week. I'm going to put you back with my receptionist."

Dr. Deyden performed surgeries on Mondays and Wednesdays, so I had to wait until the following Monday, the

27th of July. The plus side of changing the date was instead of having surgery at 3:00 p.m., I was scheduled for 9:00 in the morning. When going in for surgery, the patient is required to fast for 12 hours. A 9:00 a.m. surgery meant I would be sleeping during most of the required fast. That was the only positive point I could think of in this unexpected change of events. This setback was merely a matter of days, but it seemed like a century longer. It would mean five more days before I could return to teach school. Flexibility is not one of my stronger traits. I wasn't happy with the need to alter the dates for surgery and it was another annoying reminder that I was losing control of my life. It wasn't until my breasts were gone that I realized I missed the most important aspect of waiting for surgery. I had my breasts one extra week.

When I joined Brittany in the store to see how she was doing, I randomly picked up an expensive purse and walked over and bought it. I didn't even need a new purse. The hasty purchase was so unlike me but I ended up using it for several years. That purse was a reminder of how quickly things can change when you're dealing with cancer and it represented that I still had control over some things in my life, little as they may be.

I wasn't apprehensive about the second biopsy, scheduled for my right breast. The biopsy on my left breast went smoothly and I expected this experience to be the same. Dr. Deyden's office arranged the appointment at the only location with an opening that fit my time constraint. My daughters Julie and Kimberly accompanied me, after which we planned to go out to lunch together. It was nice having them along and we visited about Kimberly's desire to participate in the 60K Susan G. Komen Breast Cancer walk in the fall. She was passionate about it and I could see it was her way of doing something constructive. I think my children felt helpless with my situation and I marvel how each found their own creative way to handle it.

When the time came for my biopsy, I changed into another paper gown and walked into the appointed room. Was I beginning to feel more comfortable in these gowns? At least I could remember the opening was in the front. The doctor entered the room and explained the procedure which was different from my previous biopsy. As the technician searched for the designated spot on the ultrasound, I was given a shot of Lidocaine. Before the numbing could take effect, the biopsy was preformed immediately and quickly, with pain that wasn't necessary. The doctor then implanted a small metal device in my right breast so the surgeon could locate the spot during surgery. As I dressed, I wondered if maybe they wanted to hurry with the procedure so they could go to lunch. Whatever the case, it was a completely different experience than my first biopsy and I wondered how that doctor would feel if she came to Randy's office for dental work and he began before the numbing took effect.

Waiting for the results of this biopsy was nothing compared to the first biopsy, which disclosed the likelihood of cancer. We had decided on a bilateral mastectomy anyway, so it was basically information that would assist my doctor in surgery. Dr. Deyden did take the time to call and report that the mass in my right breast consisted of precancerous cells.

He summed up simply with, "It is just a matter of time and cancer would have invaded your right breast as well."

The mammogram on the right breast had come back normal, just like the left breast had been the previous year. If I did not remove the right breast, I would be facing surgery again, possibly followed by more rounds of chemo. I definitely wanted to travel this road only one time and was grateful for my doctor's wisdom and foresight. The decision to remove both breasts was validated and I would never have to wonder if we did the right thing.

The week before surgery also found me at the hospital to pre-register. This alleviated a lot of paper work the day of surgery, and helped me know what to expect and where to go. I sat across the desk from a very friendly woman who asked the necessary questions and had me sign multiple pieces of paper. We chatted lightly and as I left she remarked on my positive attitude despite having a diagnosis of cancer and being scheduled for a double mastectomy. I remember being surprised, not expecting to act any different. In retrospect, I think I was in a state of denial at times and my mind didn't process all that was happening. I was a casual spectator, removed as far away as possible from the authenticity of my situation. It was my current approach to coping.

There were times when reality would confront me head on. I remember one evening Randy and I went to a movie. It was a romance/comedy and it completely distracted me from all that was on my mind. However, as the movie ended and the credits crossed the screen, I was completely engulfed with anxiety and sorrow. I cried all the way home. I tried to determine the cause for this senseless reaction. It was probably the first time I had gone for two hours without thinking about cancer and my mind was paying me back for attempting to escape. When I returned to reality, it was a powerful jolt. Good thing it wasn't a sad movie.

There is a positive side to everything and I generally try to look for it after getting over the disappointment. Having to postpone my surgery would give me a few more days to prepare. More time to get ready for the school year I wouldn't get to start; more time to help Brittany get ready for her senior year of high school; and more time to get my house clean for the lengthy dry spell it would be facing. Grocery shopping and laundry were added to my to-do list and before long I could see the wisdom in having a few more days. By now you've probably figured out I'm a "prepared freak".

My husband had different ideas about how the extra time could be well spent. He reserved a room at a brand-new Hilton in a neighboring town so we could have a little vacation and quality time together. I will be forever grateful that he whisked me away for a much-needed break from all the stress of preparing for a surgery and subsequent chemo. It was another opportunity to escape reality. He planned it for the weekend right before surgery and so I adjusted my huge list of things to accomplish and left undone what wasn't all that important anyway. Thank goodness for a husband who could see past the mundane, unnecessary trivia that often cluttered my life.

I remember thinking it seemed funny to be staying in a hotel just a few miles from our home. I didn't realize it then, but this little escape would become a cherished memory to add to our love story. As we entered the glossy polished tiled reception area, I reflected on the events that led us to our wedding day thirty-six years earlier.

Before we met, Randy and I attended two separate universities, making it rather a miracle that we even crossed paths. We actually didn't until the summer after my junior year. I had successfully made it through three years at Brigham Young University without getting married. It wasn't that I didn't have opportunities, but I was holding out, always giving the excuse that I wanted to finish my education. That was a half-truth. I hadn't found the right guy.

Returning home to Arizona from college each summer found me following the same routine. First, I would madly look for a job, which would be hard to find for a short three months. It didn't take me long to hook up with my old friends and we would begin the search for activities and dances, hoping to meet some new faces. Laura, one of my high school friends, was up to date with the latest. I would deliberate with her about our summer plans, which of course included available young men.

I clearly recall the warm June night I asked Laura, "Do you know the name of the boy who was with Janet last night?

He is tall with thick blond hair. Is he dating her? His last name starts with a B, but it's different and hard to remember."

Laura looked at me skeptically and replied, "You must mean Randy Bretzing. He is super quiet and rarely dates. He's very committed to school. I know he's majoring in chemistry and I heard he's applying to dental school. Don't waste your time. Not much opportunity there."

The good news was that he was available. I could work around the "quiet and rarely dates" part. Loving a challenge, I silently vowed to make sure he noticed me. I had to work fast with a limited time line of summer vacation.

My first opportunity came on the second Saturday in June. A group of college students had organized a tubing trip down the Salt River, located about twenty miles from Arizona State University where we were meeting. Laura had already dictated my role that day – I was to accompany her in the same car as Alex, a boy she wanted to impress. I don't know why I agreed to that, except I didn't have any better options at the time. As we were gathering the inner tubes for the float and loading the cars, that "tall, blond" guy I referred to earlier appeared on the scene. Just seeing Randy up close caused me to drop the tube I was holding and gawk. In fact, I was so mesmerized I couldn't get my mouth to move when he asked,

"Does anyone need a ride to the river?"

Before I could regain function of my vocal chords, he was gone. My only hope was that he would float down the river in my group. As luck would have it, I never saw him again that day, making the trip, in my eyes, a total flop.

Hoping to recover quickly from my first thwarted attempt to meet Randy, I attended a dance the following weekend. As I entered the large room, I scanned the crowd for any signs of him. I was in luck. There he was, clear across the dance floor, casually chatting with friends. Now I had to come up with a way to make myself visible, which for me was not an easy task.

I was innately shy which was luckily counter-balanced with a large dose of determination.

As I slowly made my way to his area, my path was intersected by an intruder who asked me to dance. I couldn't believe it. Didn't he see I was on a mission and dancing was a mere interruption? Being the polite person I am, I accepted and tried to carry on a casual conversation, keeping an eye on Randy who was still laughing and visiting with his friends. When the song finally ended, I quickly excused myself and resumed my hunt.

I had almost reached my target, when Randy walked over to a girl and asked her to dance. The positive was he did dance. The negative was the girl he chose was adorable and they were engaged in an animated conversation, obviously enjoying each other's company.

I decided to strike up a conversation with some of the group he was with, hoping that he planned to return. After the song ended, I noticed him making his way back and before I knew it, he was a mere three feet away. Trying not to appear obvious, I continued chatting with those around me, probably talking a bit louder than necessary so my presence wouldn't be overlooked. My attempt at being charming worked, but not with the one for which my efforts were intended. Other boys in the group asked me to dance and it wasn't until the end of the evening that I finally got my chance with Randy. He asked me to join him on the dance floor for the last dance of the night, which turned out to be the first dance of our summer courtship.

Once Randy discovered me, the attraction was mutual and we spent the summer getting to know each other. I was confident I had met the man I wanted to marry and I proceeded to win his heart by way of his stomach. I made him delicious desserts, his favorite being my signature strawberry pie. He asked me out every free moment he had and we never tired of talking and sharing our dreams. When it was time for us to resume our studies at different universities, we were faced with the dilemma of how to proceed with our relationship. We were both smitten and neither wanted to be satisfied with just a summer romance. To keep me out of circulation, Randy gave me his fraternity pin and with promises to write, we parted. But not for long.

Did I mention that Randy loved football? When ASU played BYU in Provo that fall, Randy felt it was an opportune moment to see a good game and visit me. I'm still not sure which was first on his list, the game or me. It didn't really matter, because he used that occasion to ask me to marry him. It probably wasn't the most amorous proposal or worthy of a romance novel—in the parking lot of my apartment building after the game was over—but to me it was beautiful in every way. I had found the man of my dreams, and he had found his "Pixi", the term he lovingly gave me and has used to this day.

After graduating in Early Childhood Education that following summer, I secured a teaching job in a large school district in Mesa, Arizona. Just two short months after I began the school year, Randy and I were married, confusing my students with the last name change. Some never adjusted and just called me "Teacher" all year.

As dreamy as our wedding day was, it was not free of challenges. After the ceremony, the axle on Randy's car broke on the way to the wedding luncheon. It was the only transportation we owned, and our means to go on our honeymoon. The morning after our wedding day found Randy under the car fixing it, instead of proceeding on our already too short honeymoon. Fortunately, Randy's Mom came to the rescue and loaned us her car, not having confidence in the reliability of our old clunker.

Our honeymoon was simple, but lovely. We spent a short weekend at a family cabin, coming back to the valley to watch an ASU football game on Saturday night. Previously, Randy had won student tickets on the fifty-yard line for the Washington State game and it happened to fall on our honeymoon weekend. He couldn't bear to give up such amazing seats, and I had learned early in our courtship his love for the game. It was the first event we attended as husband and wife and I was glowing with pride to be in public, by his side. After an exciting win, we drove back to the cabin that very evening, anxious to return to our romantic hideout in the pines.

I was quickly brought back to the present as Randy escorted me into a beautiful room that was ours for the night. It was quite different than the rustic honeymoon cabin, but the characters were the same, as well as the plot. As lovely as our time together was, our escape ended all too soon. The drive home was silent as we returned to the harsh reality of surgery and the permanent loss of both my breasts the next day.

After learning I had cancer, I never knew what to expect when it came to my emotions, so for the most part I hid them when I could. There was so much to do before facing my surgery that I kept myself busy with trivial matters. I didn't have a lot of time to think about what was going to happen in just a few days, or perhaps I didn't want to think about it. Maybe not thinking about it was my way of coping with the future while trying to remain cheerful and optimistic. I developed a file in my mind which I labeled "Cancer" and I swiftly shoved all information that I couldn't handle quickly inside to review later, someday. I viewed this experience as a brief interruption in my otherwise "normal" life, having no doubt that after surgery and four to six quick rounds of chemo, I'd resume the life I had always known.

*July 29, 2009*

*Dear Journal,*

*This day has been full of so many emotions, the most intense being the removal of the gauze bandages wrapped around my chest. Along with the yards of gauze discarded into the garbage went my last thread of ridiculous hope that my breasts were not really gone. Like a ghost, I can actually feel they are there, but when I look down, they have disappeared.*

3

# SURGERY

No matter how we try, we can't stop time. The 27th of July came. As I look back on this day, I wonder how I remained so calm. I was about to permanently lose both of my breasts. My desire to rid my body of the enemy was the motivation that drove me to this point. I really didn't have a choice when it came to surgery as the cancer would continue to spread and invade other areas of my body. So, instead of mourning my loss, I tried to focus on the positive. I was grateful that something could be done to prolong my life and rid me of this foe.

Even though it was barely sunrise, the Arizona morning was typically warm and humid. Randy carried my small bag to the car and we solemnly began the twenty-minute drive to the hospital. I envied the rush hour traffic, wishing I was as anxious to get to my destination. I kept close tabs on my thoughts so my mind wouldn't go places I couldn't handle. Looking out the window, I concentrated on the scenery, casually mentioned the weather to Randy, and rehearsed in my mind what I had packed for the hospital. *Did I remember to tell Lori to make extra booklets for the first day of school? I wonder if Randy remembered to feed the dog before we left home.* As we neared the hospital, it was more difficult to control my thoughts and for a minute I thought I was going to throw up.

Entering the hospital parking lot, Randy asked if I wanted to be dropped off near the entrance while he parked the car. Not wanting to wait alone, I declined. Walking together into Registration, we sat and waited our turn to sign some final paperwork. Next to us in the small waiting area was a little boy, about three years old, innocently playing with a few toys brought from home. I wondered if he was the one having surgery that day. He didn't seem to have a care in the world. Oh, to be as a little child!

My name was finally called and I hurried over and signed a paper after showing the secretary my insurance card and picture ID. Randy and I were told directions to the surgical floor, most of which I couldn't follow, so I was glad my husband was there to get me to the right place.

After checking in at the surgical desk, I was greeted by a cheerful nurse who took my vitals and then handed me a bag for my belongings. I was instructed to take everything off and put on the folded blue hospital gown and socks. As he closed the bathroom door behind me, I panicked. I couldn't remember if the ties on the gown went in the front or the back. When spouting off the long list of memorized directions, he talked so fast that my brain was at least one sentence behind.

I quickly stuck my head out the door before he got away and blurted, "Where do the ties go again?"

I don't know why this is such an issue for me, but I think it stems from wanting to get things right. Oh well, the gowns are "one size fits all" and by the time I got it on and wrapped it around so I was half way modest, the ties ended up on my left side anyway.

Being alone in the bathroom gave me a sobering moment to think. I was about to take the first step in ridding my body of cancer. It would be a relief to have the enemy removed, but at the cost of losing both breasts. How quickly my life had changed in just five weeks. Instead of the wonderful plans I had made for my summer, I was now in a hospital bathroom, a victim of CANCER. Cancer was the last thing I ever expected to face in my lifetime. I guess most of us are so busy with living that we never really think about how we might die.

I stared at my reflection in the large mirror above the bathroom sink. Staring back was a fifty-eight-year-old body that had betrayed me. Hadn't I taken excellent care of it, never partaking of harmful substances and watching what I ate? I often received comments about how much younger I looked than my birthday candles revealed. It amazed me how cancer could silently tip-toe in and create unseen havoc on its prey before being discovered. Without an invitation, it had taken up residence and now I was kicking it out. Hopefully, for good.

I had already spent too much time in the bathroom and soon someone would be knocking on the door to see if I was alright. Shoving my thoughts aside, I mentally reviewed the nurse's instructions and tried one more time to empty my bladder. I couldn't think of anything worse than having to pee after my IV was started. I've learned since that it's not a big deal. The IV pole just goes right along with you, wherever you need to travel. Carefully folding my clothes, I methodically placed them in the plastic tie bag with my name written in black marker, and exited the bathroom. There was no spring in my step.

I was accompanied to a little cubicle and told to lie on the bed. A kind nurse brought pillows and made me as comfortable as possible. My favorite was the heated blanket she offered that helped alleviate the chill. Having had six children and two previous surgeries, I knew the next step would be to start an IV. I'm always thankful when this part is over, hoping for an experienced nurse that can accomplish the task on the first attempt. I have been a recipient of both ends of the spectrum when it comes to skill at inserting the needle.

I soon found I was in for more than a needle in my arm. A nurse came in and told me he was there to put dye in my breasts so the lymph nodes would show up during surgery.

How would you like getting a shot in each tender breast? No one prepared me for this. My anxiety over the matter doubled when I saw the needle. It had to be half a foot long. Luckily, it was impossible to watch the procedure in my position and the pain was over quickly. Now I just had to wait for the IV which seemed simple in comparison. The nurse was an expert and got it in place correctly the first time. I was finally able to relax, knowing that the worst of what I would be able to remember was over.

Now all I had left to do was wait for my turn for surgery, which while lying on a hospital bed seems like centuries. My husband and I engaged in light conversation, both of us avoiding the topic of the impending loss. Before we had a chance to endure painful lags in the conversation, a nurse poked her head past the drawn curtain and informed me that my mom had arrived. I told the nurse to send her in.

My dear, sweet Mom. How difficult this had to be for her. Mom was the hardest to tell and I put it off as long as I could, so she ended up being the last to hear of my cancer diagnosis. I knew she would worry and I hated to drag her through more sorrow. We had both been witnesses to breast cancer taking the life of my aunt, her last days being painful and grueling. My mom had a recent brush with death herself, having spent a week in ICU earlier that year. She wasn't in the best of health and I didn't want to be the one to add to her burdens, but here she was as only a mom would be, supporting me in my hour of need.

I thought of the stories my mother shared about my birth. I was born on a beautiful spring morning in May, just in time for her to be honored for the first time on Mother's Day. The most prominent feature she noticed was the dimple in my chin, which has yet to be carried forward by any of my posterity.

She was a devoted, loving mother who too early became a single mom trying to handle double responsibilities. My dad deserted us both before I celebrated my first birthday. My memories revolve around the dad who adopted and raised me from the time I was four. My parents were not able to have more children, leaving me an only child. Despite my constant longing for the company of siblings, I had a wonderful childhood growing up in a home full of love and encouragement. My dad passed away about five years ago, but my mom continued being a constant in my life, always willing to listen and share her nuggets of wisdom as I raised my own family. I couldn't ask for a better, more loving mother, and despite the hardship it would be for her to sit and wait through my surgery, she wasn't about to miss it.

The three of us visited until my surgeon, Dr. Deyden, finally arrived. It was reassuring to see his familiar face and I learned he had a sense of humor that morning. He was quickly explaining the surgery and mentioned something about another doctor doing such and such which quickly caught my attention. I panicked and asked him if he was still doing my surgery. He turned around, looked behind him and grinned, saying,

"Yes, I'm the only doctor here."

I tried to explain my confusion and he realized that the "other doctor" he referred to was the anesthesiologist, who of course I would want on the team. I was relieved to know I was in good hands and I relaxed. When the "other doctor" walked in, he smiled and explained what he would be doing but before he finished, I was out.

The next thing I remember was hearing my name, but I didn't want to respond. I wanted to go back to sleep. I drifted off again, only to be startled by loud annoying voices. If I kept my eyes closed, maybe they would leave me alone. When I heard nurses firmly giving instructions in energetic voices, I became conscious of where I was. Realizing the voices were addressing me, I reluctantly opened my eyes. I was told someone was here to see me. It was a visit from my friend, Dr. Burton. He had been performing surgery that morning and had stopped by to see how I was doing. I remember thinking how nice it was of him to come by, and then drifted off to sleep again.

When I awoke, I was being pushed into an elevator, probably on the way to my room. I heard my uncle speaking, insisting that they could all fit in the elevator and ride together. I was glad I didn't have to worry about settling the issue and must have fallen asleep again since I don't remember getting off the elevator. I woke up as I realized they wanted me to get into another bed. The next thing I knew I was in my hospital bed but have no memory how I got there. I finally became aware enough to comprehend that I was supposed to remain awake, so I gave up and tried to cooperate with the nurse's instructions.

Everyone is so busy in a hospital with responsibilities to perform while the patient would prefer being left alone to rest. I had to remember that this was their job and I should be glad they were excited about doing it. One of the nurses raised the head of my bed, which suddenly brought on nausea. I mentioned this and was immediately given something in my IV. Thankfully it worked quickly and the feeling passed. I didn't feel much pain but was aware of the thick gauze bandage tightly wrapped around my chest, where my breasts should be. The damage was done and they were gone, the task accomplished while I was unconscious and couldn't change my mind. I smiled inwardly as I imagined a scene with me protesting right before they were taken. "Wait! Wait! Let me think about this a little longer!" I wondered what actually happened to my breasts after being removed. Were they just tossed in the garbage?

The rest of the day in the hospital was a blur. I kept drifting in and out of a restless sleep, only to awaken to see someone trying to visit with me. Although I wasn't very responsive, I was grateful for the thoughtful friends and family who took the time to drop by.

The visit I remember the most that day was from Dr. Deyden. His five foot eight stature and accompanying grin seemed to appear suddenly at the end of my bed. He explained what he had found during my surgery. The lymph nodes on my left side had been removed because the primary node had cancer. After being sent to the lab, a total of four lymph nodes were positive for cancer. With the lymph nodes absent under my left arm, I would not be able to use that arm for blood pressure, IVs or blood draws for the rest of my life.

I asked him again if chemo would be necessary, as if by magic the answer would change if I asked enough times. He assured me I would need four to six treatments. I inquired when it would start and was relieved to hear that it wouldn't be for at least a month, giving me ample time to heal. With the dreaded chemo safely in the future, I could put it out of my mind, at least temporarily. He also informed me he had ordered a CT scan and a bone scan to be done during my hospital stay. I was too worn out to ask why and just nodded my head in agreement.

Before Dr. Deyden had a chance to move on to his next patient, I went back to the subject of my upcoming chemo and shot out the most pressing question about my impending future, "So where do I go for the next phase of my treatment?"

"Well, there is a cancer clinic right next to this hospital. The doctors are exceptional and I highly recommend them."

"Which doctor should I make an appointment with? Will you help me pick the best one in the group?"

"You couldn't go wrong with any of these doctors. They are all highly qualified."

"I'm sure they are, but I want the BEST one." In my present state, I felt justified in being a little picky.

Not responding, he gave me a big grin and left the room. I felt safe with this surgeon and was relieved he had referred me to Desert Oncology, the name of the cancer clinic next to the hospital. It brought me peace of mind to have a place to go for whatever treatments would be necessary. I trusted Dr. Deyden enough to proceed with his recommendation, feeling no need to shop around. I didn't have the energy to do so anyway.

It was nice to have Randy with me throughout the day, but even attentive husbands need to eat and sleep so I reluctantly said good-bye for the evening. My first night was typical of life in a hospital. As soon as I would doze off, I was suddenly aware of another presence in the room checking my vitals and IV bags. Since my son-in-law is a nurse who works the night shift, I was more tolerant of these procedures and the necessity for night nurses to perform their jobs.

By the next morning I was ready to eat something. I waited with anticipation, but no one arrived with a breakfast tray. When I finally asked the nurse about my breakfast, she informed me that I needed to fast before the CT scan. That was bad news since I didn't remember eating much of anything the day before and I was starving.

Since I wasn't going to be allowed the one thing I looked forward to that morning, I tried to busy myself with a magazine between having more blood drawn and my vitals taken. Finally, someone came to transport me for the CT scan and I was wheeled off to another location. I was uncomfortably aware of the different stares coming from non-patients as I was pushed down the halls of the hospital. I minimized my embarrassment by closing my eyes most of the way, especially in the elevator, and so had no idea where I was when I arrived for the scan.

Before I knew it, I was lifted onto a thin table, with the IV hook-up following me like a shadow. I was told that a substance would be injected into my veins that would cause my lower body to feel very warm. Sometimes patients thought they were urinating but I was to rest assured I was not, and to ignore the sensation. I was instructed to hold perfectly still while pictures were taken before and after the substance was given. I asked if I could listen to my iPod during the procedure and was given permission. During my vacation in Utah I had purchased an iPod for this very purpose. I knew I would be facing multiple tests and possibly hours of chemo so I figured music would provide a welcome distraction and help pass the time.

When the CT scan was over, I was wheeled back to my room where visitors were waiting. It was so nice to see my friend Peggy and my youngest daughter, Brittany. They were the first familiar faces I had seen that day and I was thrilled to have them around to pass the time and share some laughter. Even though it hurt to laugh, it was truly medicine for the soul.

We had just barely begun visiting when another woman walked in from "Face in the Mirror" wanting to give me a facial. She saw I had company and said she would return. I told her not to forget, because I definitely wanted to receive the benefits of her services. Not long after, another woman came and introduced herself as a social worker. The morning was getting busy. I was a little perplexed why the staff thought I needed a social worker, but I politely listened while she explained the various services the hospital and cancer center offered and was grateful for the bulging bag of materials she brought for reference and my use.

The social worker asked about my plans for chemo and if I had chosen an oncologist yet. I told her I planned to use the Banner Desert Cancer Center next to the hospital and she applauded my choice. She then asked if I had picked a doctor within the group and I asked her if she had any recommendations. She seemed pleased to help me out in that department, singling out two. Dr. Jensen was older and very experienced; Dr. Polowy was young, but also very capable. However, Dr. Polowy was known to spend plenty of time with his patients, never causing them to feel rushed at appointments.

As I was weighing the information in my mind, Brittany spoke up and said, "Mom, you should definitely go with the one that spends more time with you."

I quickly agreed, making a mental note of his name so I could request him when I saw my surgeon again. I thanked the social worker for the helpful bag of information and gifts and for taking the time to stop by. Pausing a moment to glance in the bag, I pulled out a heart shaped pillow. The woman explained that volunteers made these for mastectomy patients to bring comfort while healing. As I placed it under my arm, it immediately relieved the aching and pressure I was experiencing. I used that pillow for months following surgery and wished I could've personally thanked the sweet person who took the time to make it. A few years later, I traced my pillow and made a pattern, making similar pillows for others facing this physical and mental challenge.

I was surprised by the unexpected visitor and her concern for me. I didn't realize at the time how much I would need the information she brought as well as the services provided by the hospital. Like the cancer file in my mind, I had Brittany place the bag in the corner of my room, not wanting to take the time to read the copious amounts of information.

Somewhere during all the visiting, I must have eaten some lunch, but I don't remember. It seemed like I was pretty busy for someone who was in a hospital bed recovering from surgery. Nurses and lab technicians were coming in and out along with others making their rounds. Between the interruptions I was trying to visit with friends which ended suddenly when they whisked me off for my bone scan. Again, I had to endure the tortuous ride through the hospital halls, hoping I didn't see anyone that might possibly know me. Without my routine shower and opportunity to get ready for the day, I had no idea how poorly I must have looked. At least I felt good enough to still care.

This time I ended up in what was probably the basement with its cold, bare walls. I was wheeled into another room with a huge tube like the one used for my CT scan earlier that morning. I asked again if I could listen to my iPod during the scan and was granted permission. Upon being lifted on another flat, hard table, I was instructed to hold perfectly still. The whole scan took about twenty minutes after which I was wheeled from the room and left among a row of empty beds in the dimly lit basement. I was told that someone from transportation would be coming to take me back to my room shortly.

Maybe it was the cold atmosphere of the basement, or perhaps the lack of having other people around, but I suddenly felt warm tears running down my face. *What was I doing here anyway? Why did they have to run all these tests?* I hadn't expected this and it frightened me. I wished I had asked questions when Dr. Deyden informed me of the imaging scheduled for the day after surgery.

I'm sure the wait was shorter than it seemed and when the young man came to wheel me back to my room, I was embarrassed to have him see me cry. I quickly got myself back together and by the time I was in my room and around other people, I had returned to my upbeat, positive self. I pushed the feelings aside, not wanting to deal with them, excited to visit more friends and family who had arrived since I was gone.

I was happy to see the lady from "Face in the Mirror" return to give me a facial. I agreed to have her go ahead and do it even though friends and family were in the room. She made me feel beautiful despite my condition and then presented me with a lovely embroidered bag full of cosmetics and lotions. I was surprised to see they were top of the line products and was grateful for those who took the time to serve. I hope these organizations realize how much assistance they provide for women going through a life changing experience. It was a highlight of my hospital stay and the products were used and appreciated for many months. Everyone was so supportive and kind and it warmed my heart to see others spend personal time to make my adjustment easier.

The family and friends who could come and see me in the hospital made the day fly by and before I knew it I was facing my second night. Tomorrow I would get to go home and finish recovering in the comfort of familiar surroundings. I was exhausted from my busy day and actually slept well. The nurses didn't bother me as much as the night before.

The next morning brought another visit from my surgeon. He wanted to see me before checking out as well as give instructions on incision care and making future appointments. During surgery, three drains were placed that needed to be emptied several times a day. I had two on the left side where cancer was found, and one on the right. Nurses had emptied the plastic bottles during my hospital stay, but now I was trained in the proper way to empty them and deal with their presence during showers and sleeping. I could see how they would appear to be a little bulky under clothing and asked how long I would need them. I was told about a week, depending on how much fluid was still draining from my incision. A greater question in my mind was how they were going to be removed as each container was connected to a tube inserted under my skin. I was told the drains would be pulled out in the office when they were no longer needed. I doubt if that could be accomplished without some measure of pain. After all I had already experienced, I was still somewhat of a wimp when it came to needles and pain.

Dr. Deyden explained that as soon as I arrived home, I could remove the wide gauze that was wrapped around my chest. Why didn't they just remove it at the hospital? Probably because they didn't want patients freaking out when they found out their breasts were really gone and they were totally flat. This reality was best handled in the privacy of one's home. I wondered how I would react when the time actually came.

I was given paper work with a prescription for pain along with instructions for self-care spelled out in writing. I'm glad they do this because I'm sure I'm not the only patient who struggles to remember all the verbal directions. As the doctor left, he mentioned that I was somewhat anemic and suggested a few things to eat to help remedy that situation.

Even though I had been in the hospital a short time, I had grown attached to Marianne, a friendly, caring nurse assigned to the day shift. Her presence and cheerful smile always brightened the whole room and she never seemed to be in a hurry. I felt she was there just for me and I sensed an understanding that some nurses didn't seem to have or take time to show. She asked if I had chosen an oncologist yet, and was pleased to hear it would be Dr. Polowy. He was clearly a favorite among the hospital staff. That was a good sign and I was thankful for additional confirmation that I had chosen the right specialist to handle my cancer.

I was going to miss Marianne and saddened that this would be our last morning together. My bed would be empty, but for only a short time as another would take my place to occupy her time and be the recipient of her compassion. I felt fortunate to have had such a capable, caring nurse to assist me during my three-day stay.

When Randy arrived for a short visit before returning to work, Marianne suggested I take a walk with his help around the hospital floor. It felt good to get out of bed, but I was weak and shaky and glad to have Randy's support. We walked down a hallway close to my room that had various colorful paintings. As I got closer I noticed they were contributed by cancer patients. Each painting was accompanied with a narrative, explaining the symbolism of the artwork and the artist's feelings about their journey with cancer. I was mesmerized by every story and painting and my eyes began to open to the unique road I was about to travel. The paintings spoke for themselves and even though done by amateurs, the messages of the brush strokes touched me deeply. As I read each narrative, tears came to my eyes and I mourned for each cancer victim. Some wrote of cancer recurring, while others shared the trauma of being diagnosed with more than one type of cancer. I couldn't handle the thought of either of these possibilities.

I became tired of standing and told Randy we needed to go back to my room. I'm not sure if it was as much physical fatigue as it was the powerful impact of the art work and accompanying stories. To be honest, even though I was putting up a good front, I was terrified and I shuddered to think of my cancer spreading or not being cured. Although the stories were inspiring, I was awakened to the possibility of cancer's cruel potential.

As we approached where we had begun the morning's walk, I noticed that in the room next to mine was an elderly woman wearing a scarf tightly tied around her head. She was sitting at the side of her bed with her thin, bony legs hanging down. I looked away quickly—I didn't want to stare—but just seeing her sad countenance caused a lump to form in my throat. I felt so badly for her and yet, this was the world I was entering. I didn't want to be a part of it. I wanted nothing to do with scarves, hats, or wigs. It shook me as I thought that in the near future, I would also need to cover my head to hide my baldness. I didn't want to look like I had cancer. Was that even possible?

Again, I forced the emotions that were about to surface to the furthermost corner of my mind. I couldn't think about that now. Thank goodness I returned to a room with talkative friends and succeeded for the moment in sweeping away the daunting scene I had just witnessed. To this day I can still clearly visualize the woman in the room next to mine. I sometimes see myself sitting down right beside her, not being able to tell the two of us apart.

After my visitors left, I lay alone in the hospital bed, with nothing to do but wait to be discharged. I wanted to forget the events of my morning walk so I ran as far away from the present as possible, allowing my mind to drift to carefree childhood days.

Even as a child, I was an over achiever which to this day still defines and shapes how I manage my time. I can't remember a moment in my life when I was bored because I always had some marvelous idea stewing in my head. Time was always an enemy because there was never enough of it to accomplish my many plans. My mom would be wearied from watching me try to fit more in a day than was humanly possible, but I never learned to adjust. I simply tried harder.

My mind first took me to my grandmother's front yard which was always a happy place for me. For several years, we lived in a small apartment attached to the back of her house and I was familiar with every inch of that yard. She had a flower bed by the front door and that small plot was one of my favorite places to play. I was fascinated by the different varieties of plants. Tall stocks and small white daisies were what I remember, but my fondest memories were made after Grandma watered. The flower bed was my kitchen and the mud created from watering was whatever meal I was preparing for the day, decorated with rocks, seeds, and a few withered flowers.

As a child, I spent a lot of time in trees. I loved to climb two particular trees in front of my grandmother's house. Each had a fork near enough to the ground to get one foot in and a branch low enough to grab and pull myself up. From there I made my way as high as I could safely go. Once comfortably in place, I watched the world below. I was an expert daydreamer. Sometimes I imagined an entirely different life, enriched with travel to distant and exotic places. Unseen in my leafy hideout, I lost track of time, completely happy to be alone and away from reality.

When I wasn't climbing trees, I was perfecting my game of jacks. My grandmother's living room had a smooth cement floor, just right for the many variations of this childhood game. I was proficient with "pat, cherry, pat", "falling star", and "pigs in the pen". If jacks had been an Olympic event, I'm sure I would've been a contender considering the many hours I devoted to honing my skills. While boys anxiously waited for recess to play ball, the girls in my class at William T. Machan School sat in dresses (required attire for the late 1950's) on the hot sidewalks playing jacks. I was a top competitor and many tried to unsuccessfully break my record.

As soon as I learned to read, I discovered the captivating world of books. I preferred reading over watching TV and once made a goal of reading every single book in my elementary school library, beginning on the first shelf moving right. I abandoned that goal when I realized that each week other students were checking out books and there was no way I could keep track of my progress. That didn't keep me from devouring everything I could get my hands on.

One of my favorite series was about a nurse named Sue Barton: *Sue Barton, Student Nurse*; *Sue Barton, Cruise Nurse*; *Sue Barton, Rural Nurse*. I read them all and decided at a young age I was going to be a nurse. It took some years to realize that I wasn't cut out for a career in nursing. I couldn't bear to see anyone suffer, the sight of blood nauseated me, and I had a personal aversion to needles. I loved reading about nursing, but when it came to doing, teaching was my forté. As a young girl, I would come home from school and set up my own pretend classroom. When I couldn't get my friends to sit and listen to my lessons, I would line up all my dolls, who happened to be stellar students. Discovering my real talent for teaching came as I grew to know myself, but I never lost my fascination for the nursing profession and often wonder if I could have overcome the reasons I didn't pursue that path.

During the short three days after my mastectomy, I had the best nurses a person could hope for. Marianne brought me back to the present by waltzing in and cheerfully announcing that the moment I had been waiting for had finally arrived. The paper work was complete and I was free to go. I had mixed feelings. Of course, I was anxious to get home to my own bed and surroundings, but I had already made friends on the third floor. They understood my feelings and were ready and able to answer my many questions about the road ahead. I vowed I would come back and visit the staff and they were kind enough to let me know I was welcome anytime. A few weeks after my discharge I did return, bringing Marianne a plate of fresh-baked cookies and a note expressing my gratitude for all she had done.

The discharge process had taken so long that Randy had to return to his dental office and his own scheduled patients. My friend Monica showed up to take me home. It didn't take long to gather my few belongings and as she walked next to my wheelchair, I thought about how much had occurred the last three days and how my body had changed. I was now leaving this chapter of my treatment plan to rid my body of cancer, only to enter another more formidable one. I was traveling home from the hospital where I would soon be removing the thick gauze bandage to view my chest for the first time. There was no way to escape the unveiling. This was something I had to face straight on and not file away.

As Monica drove up my driveway, I saw a handmade "Welcome" sign hanging from the white pillars across my front porch. This looked like the work of my oldest daughter Julie and her sweet children. As I walked into my entryway, my suspicions were confirmed. Besides being the welcoming committee, they had decorated my home with colorful pictures and sweet words they had written or scribbled, depending on the age of the artist. How truly wonderful it was to be home, surrounded by a loving daughter and adorable grandchildren. They visited briefly so as not to wear me out, but the time they took to come by, along with their thoughtful, colorful welcome warmed my heart. Family is our greatest treasure and if I hadn't known it before, it was confirmed over and over through the months and years that followed.

I wasn't home long before Randy returned from work. He took every opportunity between patients to come home and see how I was doing. It broke his heart that he couldn't be with me every second, but he was responsible for his own patients as well as keeping his staff working. When he set up his practice less than a mile from our house, he had no idea how handy this would later prove to be.

I asked him if he wanted to help remove the gauze bandage or would he like to defer the honors to Monica? I think he was grateful that she was willing to perform the unveiling. I could tell it would be difficult for him and noticed he walked out of the room, but was still close enough to listen. I wasn't the only one dreading what had to be done.

Being a skilled nurse, Monica gently and slowly began unwinding the gauze from around my midsection. At first she appeared a bit apprehensive, probably wondering how I was going to react. I tried to clear my mind and not think about what was transpiring. I didn't want to make this a bigger deal than it was. The gauze seemed to go on forever, but it finally came to an end and I had nothing to do but look down. I was surprised by my reaction. I giggled and exclaimed,

"This is how I looked when I was ten!"

Both Monica and Randy breathed a sigh of relief. I quickly threw on my pajama top and walked away from the mirror where we were standing, acting giddy and nonchalant. I thanked Monica for bringing me home and helping with the bandage. I got into bed, hoping that everyone would leave the room. I knew my reaction wasn't typical of my personality, and I wasn't sure how long I could conceal the swirl of emotions that swept over me. The unveiling proved to be more difficult than I anticipated, but I didn't want Randy or Monica to be concerned. Typical of my pattern for handling uncomfortable information lately, I tried not to dwell on it.

But deep down inside, I was reeling. My breasts were really gone. I was there when it happened, albeit unconscious. My mind knew, but my heart hadn't processed it. I thought back on the visits from the social worker, my doctor, the conversations with the nurses. They were all preparing me for the reality of what had occurred. No wonder I appeared to be doing so well in the hospital. I hadn't really accepted the cold, hard fact that two very dear parts of my body were no longer present. Part of my femininity was gone, soon to be joined by losing my hair. I thought of Randy. How was he taking this? It was his loss too. Holding back the gathering tears, I decided I needed to stop feeling sorry for myself. It was done and for the significant purpose of saving my life. I had to muster the energy to go forward.

Shoving my distress into the back of my mind, I snuggled with my heart pillow, pulled up the covers and closed my eyes. My attempt to escape was brief as within minutes, a kind neighbor came by with dinner, followed by phone calls from my adult children. I eagerly welcomed these diversions, putting distance between the memory of my loss and the reality of loving friends and family. How blessed I was to be surrounded by so many genuine, caring people who supported me.

Through the subsequent years when I began slipping into depression over my missing breasts, I would think about Ellen. When I neared the end of my treatments, my friend Ellen was diagnosed with a form of lymphoma cancer. She once remarked, "At least Claudia could cut off her cancer." This statement offended me at first, feeling that she was insensitive to my loss. When she lost her battle to cancer, I realized she had been right. She lost her life, but had her breasts. I lost my breasts, but had my life.

Monica offered to help empty my drains for the first few days and I quickly agreed. Being a nurse, she loved this kind of thing, and I didn't. It wasn't a pleasant sight to view the liquids that were constantly draining from my body. Since they had been emptied before leaving the hospital, she decided to come back later in the evening before I went to bed. I think the drains were a good excuse to check on me.

As far as surgeries go, a mastectomy rated low on the pain scale. I didn't suffer much and slept comfortably. I did take the pain medicine Dr. Deyden had given me which helped the first few days. I was grateful that I could take a shower the day

I arrived home. The three drains, my new companions, traveled everywhere I went and if I chose what to wear carefully, they weren't even noticeable. My surgery was Monday, July 27; I arrived home from the hospital on Wednesday, July 29 and I already had an appointment to see Dr. Deyden on Friday, July 31. When I called to make my appointment with my surgeon, I told the office receptionist I wanted Dr. Polowy for my oncologist. By the end of the week, Dr. Polowy's office had called and scheduled me for Monday, August 3. Already my life had changed drastically. I would be seeing more doctors in one week than I usually saw in a year. I was surprised to have an appointment with the oncologist so soon, but they didn't seem to be wasting time.

The first few days at home were anything but lonely. My home was frequented by caring friends who brought food, flowers, cards, and love. Throughout my year with cancer, I received countless cards in the mail, some funny, others inspiring. I saved every one and would often re-read them when times were tough. On several occasions a card would arrive in the mail on a day I was feeling low. I wondered at how that friend knew several days earlier I would need a lift. I never realized before how much a card could mean and vowed I would do the same for others. Taking the time to send a note or card seems simple, but is greatly appreciated by the recipient. It can change the course of their day and transform negative feelings into positive ones. Oh, the strength one receives when they know others are thinking and caring about them.

As far as recovering from the surgery, my first two days at home were uneventful. I felt tenderness around the incision, which ran clear across my chest and halfway under each arm. I was also numb throughout most of the surgical area, but especially under my left arm. I was curious if the numbness would eventually fade, or if it was going to be a constant reminder of my surgery. Probably even Dr. Deyden couldn't answer that question. Only time would tell.

On Friday, I had my check-up with Dr. Deyden. It was my first attempt after surgery to get ready to go anywhere and it wore me out. I was surprised at how the simple routine of showering and dressing could be so exhausting. Since I wasn't able to drive yet, Monica offered to take me to my appointment.

This was the first time I saw Dr. Deyden since I left the hospital. I felt pretty good so I expected it to be a routine visit. He gently examined the incision and seemed pleased with my progress, informing me he would probably remove the drains next week. The appointment took very little time since for once I didn't have any questions. I thanked him for the great job he had done and let him know how pleased I was with his care.

The appointment I was most anxious about was meeting my oncologist for the first time. Monica, sensing my uneasiness, volunteered to go with me for support. She even offered to come in and take notes during my appointment. Due to her medical training, she would understand more of what I would be told and be able to explain what I didn't understand. I decided to see the doctor on my own, but would invite her in when they began giving instructions about chemotherapy. Before attending this appointment, I found an old spiral notebook and wrote down as many questions as I could think of for Dr. Polowy. I knew I would only have so much time with him and I wanted to be prepared. I never forgot my friend Cindy's advice, and between each appointment I made a growing list of questions on a pad easily accessible on my night stand.

As Monica drove me to the Cancer Center on Monday, she tried to calm me with small talk. I don't remember any of it because all I could think about was the upcoming appointment. I don't know why I was so nervous, perhaps due to the fact I was approaching unfamiliar territory and the closer I got, the more I wanted to turn around. When we found the right building, we had to tell the security guard which doctor we were there to see before we could park. Desert Oncology was attached to the hospital, across the street from my surgeon's office.

When we walked through the double doors leading into the building, my sense of smell overcame all other senses. An overwhelming disinfectant odor permeated the building. I would become so familiar with this smell during the next few weeks and months, even years. As I entered those double doors months after my chemo treatments were finally completed, my stomach continued to lurch at the sterile odor that would remind me of the hours spent in this building. Smells unleash memories, pleasant and unpleasant.

Far too quickly we found Dr. Polowy's treatment suite. Monica pushed open the heavy door and walked into the waiting room. I hesitated in the doorway, quickly scanning the scene before me. I think all of us have a photo album in our minds containing snapshots of things we never forget. What I observed in the waiting room quickly uploaded into my album. As I looked over the room, I noticed all kinds of people, mostly older, a few wearing scarves, some completely bald. One was in a wheelchair, another extremely thin and pale. No one smiled or talked. The atmosphere was thick with solemnity and soberness.

My mind knew I had cancer. I just had surgery because I had cancer, but walking into the Cancer Center suddenly made it real for me. My legs felt weak as I mechanically followed Monica to the receptionist and wrote my name on the check-in roster. The girl behind the desk flashed a welcoming smile that I found hard to return. Reluctantly, I followed Monica to the only two empty seats together and sat. I knew Monica wouldn't leave no matter how much I pleaded. She was my ride home so it looked like I would be staying.

Monica continued with her futile attempts to visit with me while I bounced my leg up and down, a nervous habit. Her voice was in the background as I continued to look at the people in the waiting room. What I saw were varying results of chemo treatments. How many weeks before I fit right in? Like it or not, I was a cancer patient, joining the others in this room.

My sober reverie was interrupted when the receptionist called me to the front desk to provide insurance information. She handed me a clipboard holding a thick sheaf of papers, hastily giving instructions on how to fill them out. "Complete this page and sign at the bottom. Read and sign the next two pages. Next is your health history, followed by a privacy policy which you initial and then sign in two places. Any questions?"

I looked at her blankly and shook my head. Taking a pen and the clipboard, I returned to my seat. I was about halfway through the paperwork when I was called back to see Dr. Polowy. I told the nurse who announced my name that I wasn't finished with the pile of papers they gave me, but she smiled and said I'd have time in the exam room. Great. I was hoping to delay the inevitable first meeting with my oncologist. If I took enough time to fill out all the papers I could miss my appointment and think more about this. I felt like I was on a carousel that was spinning faster and faster and I couldn't get off. I've never liked fast rides.

Obediently I followed the nurse past the heavy wooden door that separated the waiting patients from the ones in the dungeons. My first stop was a large scale where I was instructed to stand to get my weight. It reminded me of the scales at the vet, large enough for a big dog to lie on. The digital numbers went up and down and then settled on my weight which the nurse recorded on her clipboard. I was then led to an exam room where my temperature and blood pressure were taken.

The nurse next handed me another one of those lovely paper gowns with the instructions, "Opens at the front", and I was left to change and finish my paperwork.

Since my surgery, I found it difficult to easily comply with the once simple task of changing my clothes. My arms just didn't lift and stretch like they previously did. Then there was the matter of the paper gown. It seems logical that they would make these paper contraptions small, medium, and large, but unfortunately they come in a size to accommodate the largest patient. The problem is, one size doesn't fit all because the arm holes practically went to my waist and the front could be wrapped around to the back. To complicate this small request to prepare for the doctor's exam, I was trying to juggle three drains hanging precariously from my chest. These new circumstances caused me to take a few extra minutes and I was fearful I would still be struggling and appearing flustered when the doctor walked in. Thankfully, I accomplished the task, caught my breath and returned to the paperwork I had been assigned. Before I could even focus on where I had left off, I was interrupted by a small knock and the entrance of my oncologist, Dr. Polowy.

This was a big moment for me. I knew my cancer and my life would be in this doctor's hands and I so desperately wanted to be pleased with my choice.

Dr. Polowy was young, well dressed in a shirt and tie, and had a smile that would put anyone at ease. I immediately knew I was in good hands because of the calm, confident air about him. After introducing himself, he gently took the unfinished paperwork out of my hands and helped me lie down on the exam table. As he carefully opened the gown to look at the work of my surgeon he remarked, "I'm going to call Dr. Deyden and tell him what a wonderful job he did on your mastectomy." Looking at the drain tubes, he added, "They sure have you all hooked up!"

He helped me return to a sitting position and told me I could get dressed. He would return in a few minutes to talk and as suddenly as he appeared, he disappeared. I couldn't help but think of the Wizard of Oz when Dorothy exclaimed, "My! People come and go so quickly here!".

I dressed as hastily as I was able, only to wait for what seemed like centuries for Dr. Polowy to come back. He was probably seeing another patient, but I was extremely anxious to talk about my future. Instead of completing my paperwork, I took out my notebook, going through the questions in my mind, deciding which ones were the most important. I wondered if every patient had as many questions as I did.

Upon his return and giving me his full attention, Dr. Polowy listened patiently to each of my concerns. I had countless questions, most of which couldn't be answered in one appointment.

"What caused my breast cancer?"

"I have five daughters. Do they need to have mammograms before they are 40? What's in store for them?" He listened carefully as I continued to fire more questions at him.

"What side effects can I expect from chemo?"

"What are my chances for survival?"

Some questions he answered briefly while he sat quietly through others as I released some of my anxiety. He was an expert listener and one of the first people I had talked to that seemed to really comprehend my anguish. He not only listened with his ears, but with his heart. Reflecting on this first meeting, I am amazed at the way Dr. Polowy patiently and kindly endured my barrage of questions. I could easily see why he was so highly recommended.

As I finally exhausted my present concerns, he excused himself again to go and retrieve some information that would visually help me with some of my questions.

My time alone in the exam room allowed me to organize my thoughts. I couldn't believe how fortunate I was to have an oncologist who understood my situation. I was impressed with his knowledge and experience, but even more with his ability to relate to me as a patient. I was grateful for those who, barely knowing me, took the time to recommend him. The burden of my cancer diagnosis was now shared with a competent, compassionate doctor. What a contrast from the fear I felt walking into the office an hour earlier.

When Dr. Polowy returned, he invited me to sit in a chair next to him as he began to answer my questions more completely and explain my options. He showed me a colored bar graph, printed out for my individual case. At the very top of the page was printed in bold letters, "Shared Decision Making." I liked that title. "Shared" meant that I had some say in this and I felt a return of control for the first time since I learned I had cancer. It then stated my age: "58" and my General Health as "Excellent." The next few lines gave more information which he quickly went over: "Estrogen Receptor Status: Positive; Tumor Size 3.1-5.0 cm; Nodes Involved: 4-9; Chemotherapy Regimen: Third Generation Regimen". I wondered what that meant, but didn't ask as I was anxious to hear about the colored graph.

He quickly went on to explain the bars on the graph. The first bar was titled, "Decision: No Additional Therapy". The green color indicated that if I chose not to do anything, statistics showed that in ten years, 45 out of 100 women were alive and without cancer; 51 out of 100 women would relapse, and 4 out of 100 women would die of other causes. Clearly, this was not a good choice.

The next bar was titled, "Decision: Hormonal Therapy." He explained that this was a pill taken daily for five years. If I chose this route, my chances increased from 45 without cancer in ten years to 69 out of 100. That looked a little better, but not the statistics I was looking for.

The third bar bore the title, "Decision: Chemotherapy". This one surprised me because my chances actually declined slightly from the hormonal therapy to 66 out of 100 women would be alive and without cancer in ten years.

Lastly, Dr. Polowy pointed out the final bar on the graph, titled "Decision: Combined Therapy". He explained this meant chemotherapy followed by taking the hormonal therapy for five years. In this instance, my chances of being cancer free in ten years rose to 81 percent. Taking into account the four percent who die of other causes, there was merely a 15 percent chance of my cancer returning.

I stared at the paper, trying to assimilate the information. My mind felt numb. It seemed like my thought processes were always behind and I was trying desperately to catch up. My doctor's voice faded into the background as my eyes jumped from one bar graph to another. I was immediately jolted back to the present as he went on to explain that breast cancer can spread to the liver, bones, lungs, and brain, if not treated. I will never forget the serious look on his face as he added,

"If that happens, it is not operable."

Clearly he was voting for the last bar on the graph. As nice as he was, he was not going to sugar coat what I needed to hear. Looking at the statistics, I would be foolish to opt for anything but combined therapy and my heart sank as I finally accepted the fact that chemotherapy was really going to happen. I was free to choose, but I was also accountable for my choices. The options were there as well as the consequences. My feelings of being in control were short lived. This disease had control over me and my only logical option was to accept the best treatment they had to offer and fight this disease with all the strength I had. Being informed at least allowed me to make an educated decision. After a long pause, I meekly responded, "Okay. I'm in."

As Dr. Polowy went on with more instructions, I pulled myself together and began jotting down notes.

"Chemo, every three weeks for six sessions."

"Five years of hormonal therapy (pills)";

"Blood work once a week."

"PET scan and Muga Heart scan."

Yes, there were more tests to be done. He said the office would make an appointment for a PET scan and then took the time to show me what one looked like. Any suspicious spots would show up in color, helping him to know if cancer had already spread to other areas. Since I'm a visual person, it was very helpful to see on paper what everything meant.

At this point I explained that I was a school teacher and I wondered if I could receive my treatments on a Friday and return to school on Monday. He suggested that I choose Wednesdays for treatments as the third and fourth day after chemo commonly produced the worst reactions. I would peak on the weekend and then possibly be ready to return to school on Monday.

Looking at his calendar, Dr. Polowy set a date for my first treatment. "We'll begin chemotherapy on Wednesday, August 19."

I must have heard wrong, or Dr. Polowy forgot I just had surgery because August 19 was just a little over two weeks away. I was expecting a full month to recover from surgery. When he told me he would be checking with Dr. Deyden for permission to proceed, I breathed a sigh of relief since I knew my surgeon would be on my side and insist on waiting for at least a month.

Before I could ask additional questions, a nurse entered the room whom he introduced as my trainer. Dr. Polowy then handed me some prescriptions to fill, saying he would be around at the end of my session if I had additional questions.

The nurse handed me a small booklet titled, "Chemotherapy Patient Resource Manual" and we went over some of the pages together. She pointed out the chemo drugs I would receive that bore the initials TAC and their possible side effects. I could see why they used initials for the drugs as the real names were about twenty letters long and impossible to pronounce. The day after each chemo I would be given a shot to build up my white blood cells and she went over the side effects of the shot.

Looking over the pile of prescriptions the doctor handed me, she explained the following: one was to be taken the morning and evening before and after chemo; there were two different drugs for nausea; one for diarrhea; a prescription for a cranial prosthesis (fancy name for a wig); and finally, a prescription for mastectomy bras and two breast prosthesis to take the place of what was missing.

My body and mind began to feel weary with all the information. Between Dr. Polowy and my trainer, I felt I had taken Cancer 101 in the last hour. Before the nurse could continue, I asked if Monica, who had been patiently sitting in the waiting room, could join us. She readily agreed and I felt so much better having my friend accompany me for the remainder of the appointment.

The nurse returned to my cancer notebook, showing me the numbers to call to reach the office. In most cases, I would be leaving a message and my call would be returned that day. If I needed to talk to someone right away, I could press "0". She encouraged me to call and obtain the results of my weekly blood tests as well as any scans that were performed. Next she showed me a page that listed reasons I should contact the doctor: fever over 100.5, severe vomiting or diarrhea, irregular heart beat or chest pain, dizziness or weight loss. She directed my attention to some websites I could use to obtain more information about cancer, and the names and numbers of support staff and groups that could assist me in my cancer experience. I was thrown by the phrase "cancer experience". It made it sound like some adventure or vacation. Well, it promised to be an experience alright. One that I'd never forget. Then we began the tour.

Monica and I left the exam room and followed the nurse to another section of the Cancer Center. On the way, we passed a small, narrow room where the chemo cocktails were being prepared. The nurse in this room was wearing gloves and a long-sleeved apron. On the wall hung several bags filled with clear liquid, still waiting for their assigned patient. A chill passed through my body as I viewed the contents of this room and watched the nurse concentrating on her task.

I was shown the injection room which was also small, containing one reclining chair. Here I would receive my shots. I wondered at having a room solely for the purpose of administering shots. Later, I learned the injection room was also used for any patient who may be contagious. The nurses were very careful to prevent exposing those receiving chemo to anyone who might be sick. They quickly sat you in that room until a doctor could evaluate the situation.

A few steps further led us to what was simply referred to as the Chemo Room. I quickly glanced around noticing about fifteen comfortable recliners, each next to a small table. By now, it was almost 5:00 p.m. and the room was nearly void of patients. Most had finished their treatment and gone home, reminding me of how long I had been at this first appointment. There was a nurses' station and a large refrigerator which was opened for me to inspect. It was full of various juices and drinks, which I was welcome to have during my stay. This was where I could put my lunch, but was cautioned against bringing foods with a strong odor which might cause other patients to feel nauseated. This small tidbit of information made me wonder how long a chemo session lasted. There were also crackers, cookies, and various other simple snacks. In one corner stood a closet containing blankets and pillows and I was encouraged to bring a comfortable, favorite blanket from home as the chemo room was kept cold (something I had already noted).

The nurse led me to a sign-up sheet for a program called "Look Good, Feel Better", an organization that held classes to instruct cancer patients on how to adjust make-up and hair (or the lack of it) due to the eventual effects of chemotherapy. All participants received a bag of free make-up products as well as instructions on wearing and caring for a wig, or scarves. She encouraged me to sign up right then, but I decided to wait as it was offered monthly and I wasn't quite ready to admit needing help in those areas, at least not yet.

My head was reeling with information. I had just spent about two hours learning how I was going to spend the next few months. This would be my life. It would consume my time and change my chemistry. How my body would react remained to be seen.

The tour appeared to be over as the nurse smiled and asked if I had any questions. I clutched the chemo notebook they had given me and shook my head. I wanted to ask my doctor more questions, mostly just to receive comfort, but it looked like he had already left for the day. As the nurse walked us to the door, the once filled waiting room was empty. Except for the few remaining in the chemo room, I was the last to leave. My mind felt numb as Monica drove me home and if there was any conversation, she instigated it.

I arrived home exhausted physically and mentally. What was happening to me? I wanted to get off this quickly accelerating amusement park ride and return to my previous life. I can't count how many times during my cancer journey that I thought, "I don't want to be a part of this." It was frustrating that I didn't have a choice.

I placed my chemo notebook, prescriptions, and the notes I had taken in the drawer of my nightstand, changed into pajamas, got in bed and pulled the covers over my head. I wasn't going to cry. I didn't have enough energy to cry. I just wanted to disappear. It had been a long day and I couldn't think any more about having cancer. Surely this was just a bad dream from which I would soon awake.

By the time Randy arrived home from work, I had pulled myself together and tried to explain the things I had learned at my first appointment with my oncologist. Going over the graph with him and the contents of the notebook, I regained a more positive attitude. I didn't want him to worry, and acting upbeat not only portrayed confidence and faith but it helped me as well. I reasoned that it was good to have the information I needed to proceed. Today's visit had answered a lot of questions I had about my future. I was happy with Dr. Polowy and the Cancer Center. They were organized and caring and patient with all my questions. I had to accept what was best for me and trust in their care. Really, what else could I do?

The next day I rested. After all, I was recovering from surgery and I needed to take care of myself. I visited with my children on the phone to let them know what I had learned from the visit with my oncologist. I received a call from the imaging center and was given an appointment for the PET scan. Another call scheduled the Muga Heart scan. No one was wasting time. For someone who has had very little experience with tests, scans, prescriptions, and doctors, I was feeling slightly overwhelmed. The number of appointments was increasing and it was nice having a day where I didn't have to get ready to go somewhere.

The following day was Wednesday and I had another follow up appointment with Dr. Deyden. He said he would be removing my drains which made me a little apprehensive, but they were bulky and hard to hide under clothes so it would be nice to be rid of them.

When I arrived at Dr. Deyden's office, I was called in quickly and handed another paper gown to wear. After exchanging it for my clothes, I obediently sat on the exam table waiting for my turn. I wonder if doctors realize the extent to which patients study the artwork and read the certificates on the wall while they are waiting. Unless there are magazines available, there is nothing left but to stare at the walls of the exam room. I don't know why but I rarely remembered to bring a book to read. When I did, I never brought it out because my concentration level was zero. While waiting for a doctor, I was always apprehensive and bored, but too jittery to do anything about it.

In this particular exam room, I had six different documents to read. One told a story of where Dr. Deyden had graduated from Medical school, several plaques expounded honors he had received, while yet another announced his training as a surgeon. I felt I knew just about everything I needed to know concerning my surgeon's qualifications by the time he finally entered the room.

It was good to see Dr. Deyden's familiar, jovial face that morning which immediately helped me relax. He looked at my drains and decided that only one of the three was ready to remove. The other two still had a significant amount of fluid draining into them and if they were removed too soon, this fluid would accumulate under my skin and have to be extracted with a syringe. That didn't sound too appealing so I was fine with keeping the two on my left side for a few more days. As he removed the drain on the right side he distracted me by commenting on my choice of oncologists.

"You know, there is just one thing wrong with Dr. Polowy."

Alarmed, I timidly asked, "What?"

With a grin on his face, he remarked, "He is just too good looking."

In defense of my choice, I teased, "I obviously use looks as my first criteria in choosing a doctor. I chose you, didn't I?" The concerned look on my face hadn't escaped him, though, and he laughed knowing he had me worried for a minute.

Removing the right drain wasn't as bad as I thought it would be. Dr. Deyden had a good touch and before I knew it, he had taken it out with a quick pull and covered the open wound with a bandage. He checked my incision, which was still being held together with steri-strips and said I was good to go. I made an appointment for the following Monday to remove the other two drains.

In the meantime, there was more to accomplish before the start of school. The following week was "Meet the Teacher" and I wanted to attend this event along with my substitute, Lori. I felt I owed the parents an explanation for my absence and I wanted to personally introduce Lori to the parents and children. We usually have great attendance at this event before school begins and it would be the best way to solicit the support and help of my parents.

A week earlier I prepared the families by mailing a letter explaining my absence at the beginning of the school year due to surgery. No mention had been made of my cancer diagnosis due to my principal's suggestion, but I wasn't going to try and hide it. Word had already spread throughout the neighborhood and I felt an honest approach would be best. Being visible would assure the parents I was on top of the situation. My cancer treatments would only affect me for a few months. I had already figured that with six treatments every three weeks, I would be finished before Christmas.

With Lori's help my classroom looked organized and inviting in time for the big day. Unlike previous years, I was nervous but knew how important it would be to appear confident. I had to assure each parent that their child would be in good hands and that I had chosen an amazing substitute whom I trusted and would follow the lesson plans I would prepare.

"Meet the Teacher" was scheduled just ten days following my surgery. I wore a loose top to hide the bulky presence of the two remaining drains that hung from my chest. My principal questioned my attendance at this event, but I assured her I felt fine and that it was important for me to personally reassure the parents that I had the situation under control. Did I have it under control? It's hard to say. I was certainly trying to convince everyone as well as myself that it was.

As students and parents trickled in and out that morning, I expended a lot of energy introducing Lori and providing explanations. It was often hard to read the parents' faces as I explained my unique circumstances. Most of the children were familiar with me as I have taught at the school for a number of years. They were expecting to see my face on the first day of school and I'm not sure if they understood why I wouldn't be there the first few weeks.

The two hours went by quickly, but I was totally exhausted at the completion of the morning's event. I had depleted the small amount of energy I did have trying to gain the understanding, confidence, and support of those assigned to my classroom for the year. As worn out as it made me, taking the time to meet my students and their parents before the first day of school laid a strong foundation that was invaluable in contributing to the understanding I would need that year. I outlined my condition and resulting treatment with my usual positive flair, assuring them all would be back to normal by the first of December. At least that was the plan. I hadn't had enough experience yet to know that with cancer, things rarely go as planned.

*August 25, 2009*

*Dear Journal,*

*It has been almost a week since I received my first chemo. I'm supposed to teach school tomorrow and I don't even have enough energy to get out of bed to brush my teeth. I feel like I have a bad case of the flu. If this is what it's going to be like I will never survive five more sessions. I am asking myself which is worse, the cancer or the cure?*

4

# THE FIRST CHEMO

When I received the call from Dr. Polowy's office scheduling my first chemo treatment for Wednesday, August 19, I was shocked. What happened to my full month of recovery from surgery? Apparently, Dr. Deyden had buckled and gave Dr. Polowy the green flag to begin treatment. I learned that when a surgeon and oncologist confer, the oncologist usually wins. I was certain Dr. Deyden would tell Dr. Polowy I wouldn't be ready for several weeks. To be honest, I didn't think I would ever be ready, but ready or not, the appointment was set and I didn't have much say in the matter. Dr. Polowy was anxious to get started and I trusted his judgment, despite my longing to drag my feet.

This would affect the date I planned to return to school. I had to factor in an earlier than expected chemo treatment which would cause me to miss the entire first month of teaching. In a second-grade classroom, this was the most important month, setting the tone for the whole year. It did occur to me that the sooner I started, the sooner I would finish. I got out my calendar and counted out the weeks, confirming that my ending date would be December 2nd, in plenty of time to enjoy the Christmas holidays.

During the second week of August, my daughter Kristy came from Utah with her two-year-old son, Justus, to help me following surgery. When she arrived, it was like a ray of sunshine had entered my home. I could finally take it easy and rest from the demands of preparing for school and thinking about my upcoming chemo treatments. There is nothing that takes your mind off unpleasant situations better than a toddler. I read Justus stories and enjoyed the freshness of his cheerful, childlike laugh. Having grandchildren around is the best medicine there is and the time they were with me was very therapeutic. Kristy and I had some good talks and I was able to verbalize many of my fears and feelings.

The day soon arrived for my PET scan. I was instructed not to eat anything for at least four hours before the imaging appointment. I would be given an IV in which radioactive dye would be injected into my veins. Next I would sit in a dark room for forty-five minutes at which time I couldn't visit, read or do anything to stimulate my mind, although listening to my iPod was approved. After that, I would have the scan which would take about twenty minutes. When I returned home, I wasn't to be around children or pregnant women for six hours. Kristy and Justus took this opportunity to spend the evening with other family members.

The location for the PET scan was not a familiar place so I mapped it on the internet and left in plenty of time for the appointment at 3:00 p.m. I was glad they had explained everything so thoroughly so nothing would be a surprise. Upon arriving, I was instructed to remove all my clothes and change into a long paper gown, this time with the ties in the back. Being several sizes too big, I found it hard to walk down the hallway without the back flapping open, so I was constantly grabbing the two back sections and bringing them around to the front. Those in the waiting room had an unobstructed view of the front restroom which I was asked to use before being led to a comfortable recliner. Having endured parading in public with practically nothing on, I prepared myself for my least favorite part—the insertion of the IV needle. Everything that had been explained to me on the phone transpired and before I knew it I was resting comfortably. My private cubby was dark and quiet. I leaned back in the recliner and listened to my iPod. Just as I was about to fall asleep, a nurse popped in and informed me it was time for the PET scan.

As my assigned nurse led me into the room, my eyes quickly took in the scene before me. Unlike the long narrow MRI tube, this was a wide-open tube. In front of the tube was a flat table to lie on. It was so narrow I wondered if I would fit on it without hanging over the edge. It was also very hard so I was thankful someone brought me a pillow. I was instructed to hold perfectly still and breathe normally.

As the table began to move, I decided to close my eyes so I wouldn't be aware of where I was in the tube. The table would move slowly, then stop for a period of time, then move again. My curiosity got the better of me a couple of times and I would open just one eye to see where I was. One time my upper body was in the tube, and another time my lower body. It was an interesting experience, painless and soundless. When completed, I dressed, drove myself home and spent a quiet evening with Randy.

A few days later I was scheduled to have what was called a Muga Heart scan. Again, I received an IV and a dye was injected into my veins. During this scan, I was to lie perfectly still while a camera took images of my chest. I had to change positions several times during the procedure, but again, it was very simple. I really couldn't complain about all the scans and tests they were running because not one was uncomfortable.

I asked the technician the purpose of this scan and she replied that it gave the doctor a baseline in the event my heart was affected by the chemotherapy. I had read recently that the "A" in my TAC cocktail stood for Adriamycin which could irreversibly damage the heart, even in small doses. I decided to stop reading so much.

With all these appointments to keep me busy, the night before August 19 came more quickly than I wanted. Randy had filled all my prescriptions, except the mastectomy bras and prosthesis, which I put off for nearly a year. I knew I couldn't just walk in and purchase them. I would have to arrange for fittings and I didn't have the energy to do that. Also, I wasn't quite ready to face the reality that those items were necessary.

The day before chemo, I was to take two steroid pills in the morning and two in the evening. The Monday before, I had my weekly blood test. That was all I had to do to prepare physically. My oldest daughter Julie offered to watch Justus so Kristy could be with me during my first chemotherapy treatment. As little as I wanted that day to arrive, I was thrilled to have my daughter present to offer much needed support.

Randy was deeply disappointed that he would not be the one to accompany me during my first session with chemo, as well as many of the ones that followed. Being the owner and sole dentist in his practice, his job owned him and we depended on his income. Along with the emotional concerns about my health, the strain in keeping his practice healthy compounded his worries. He kept all of his grief to himself, trying to be strong for me. Despite his brave exterior, I know he had moments of private melt downs. I often think my husband suffered more than I during our journey with cancer. Watching someone suffer is often worse than the suffering itself.

I was more anxious about my first chemotherapy appointment than my surgery. Up to this point in my life, I had taken very little medicine and chemo was designed to be strong. No one could tell me exactly how my body would react to the three different drugs dripping into my veins. The evening before chemo I was jittery and unable to focus on anything. I tried but couldn't get my mind off what I finally was required to face. Chemo was no longer in the future. It was here.

Usually before a big day, it's a good idea to get a restful night's sleep. I was not that fortunate. I couldn't fall asleep and the more I lay awake, the more frustrated I became. Finally, I sat up in bed and wrote in my journal:

*I can't sleep even though I desperately need to. In about nine hours I'll be receiving my first round of chemo. I'm just starting to feel better from my surgery and can actually function for about half of a day before crashing and needing to rest. After tomorrow, who knows how I'll feel. The list of chemo side effects runs for pages. I've read them all. I know I can't sleep because I'm scared. I don't remember ever feeling so terrified. I feel like I'm standing on a cliff and jumping into the darkness. Questions swirl through my mind. How will I react and respond to chemo? Will the cancer come back anyway? Can I still teach my second-graders and do justice to my job? Will I have the energy to carry on with my responsibilities? What will it really be like to lose my hair?*

*So many unanswered questions, but if I don't take the plunge, my life may be compromised. I must remind myself that the whole thing is in the Lord's hands anyway, so it basically comes down to trusting Him. I've done everything I can to prepare for this day. I have excellent doctors and the most amazing support group. Randy has held my hand and my heart all the way. My children are praying and cheering me on. Dear friends have brought meals, sent cards, visited, listened, and loved. I've been blessed abundantly and so I need to trust more and find the courage to press forward. I have such a big day tomorrow and I'll make things a lot easier on myself if I can get some sleep tonight.*

Having written down my emotional turmoil and the thoughts spinning in my head, I finally fell into a fitful sleep, sad to see the morning come so quickly. I woke up before the alarm, showered and dressed mechanically. I had already packed my bag containing a soft blanket, book, and iPod. At the last minute, I threw in a card game to play with Kristy. Three hours is a long time to be a prisoner to an IV line.

After a big hug and kiss from Randy, I climbed in our car, hesitant to leave the haven of our home. Over the next few years, I would travel this route countless times. The drive to the Cancer Center took about twenty minutes by freeway. On the way, I was always apprehensive and anxious, even when I knew what to expect. On the drive home, my body, mind, and emotions were numb and I was dog-tired, even though all I did was sit in a recliner. Unlike my usual chatty self, I was seldom in the mood to talk, which was hard on the person escorting me. It took copious amounts of energy to engage in conversation so I preferred to remain quiet. My friend, Lauri, understood. She was content with letting me sit silent, never attempting to make conversation. With her, it was a comfortable silence. Once when Lauri couldn't take me to get my required shot after chemo, she arranged a substitute who happened to be one of the most energetic, bubbly women I know. Normally, I love to be in her presence but the thought of riding in the car with her was so overwhelming, I drove myself.

Having my daughter with me for my initial chemotherapy was the best companion. Nervous as I was, I could be myself, and her presence was comforting. She could tell I was apprehensive, and I could tell she was worried about me. Experiencing this day together was something neither of us will forget.

When we arrived at the Cancer Center, I was handed a paper asking a few questions. The first was the most ridiculous question I had ever read.

"Do you feel like having chemo today?"

*Are you kidding? Of course I don't feel like having chemo. There will never be a day when I feel like having chemo!* I wrote something to the effect, "No, I don't. I hardly got any sleep last night and I feel nauseated." Why was I already feeling nauseous? I couldn't imagine being in a worse condition before chemo even began. Later I found that the steroid pills I took the day before were probably the reason.

The next few questions were along the line of, "Do you have a sore throat? Are you running a fever?" I had to put "No" for the remainder of the questions. I handed the questionnaire back to the receptionist, hoping my first answer would disqualify me for keeping today's appointment. I reasoned that a person should face chemo feeling strong and ready. I didn't feel ready at all, much less strong.

Apparently, no one reads the questionnaire, or they ignored my answer to question number one, because before I knew it, my name was called. The nurse led Kristy and I into the chemo room, passing the cubicle where the bulging chemo bags were being prepared and hung. I was told I could pick any chair I wished and since they were all the same, it didn't matter. I chose one near the door in case I decided to leave.

As soon as I sat down, I immediately popped back up again and asked the nurse if I could use the restroom before getting started. She smiled and showed me where it was. I was never so glad to be out of that chemo room. I didn't actually have to go to the bathroom so I just sat on the toilet and thought.

*Do I really want to go through with this?*

*Why did I buy into having chemo?*

*It wasn't too late to back out. Once the IV is in and the drugs start dripping, then it's too late.*

I wondered if anyone actually changed their mind right before they got the IV.

*It will take just one chemo treatment for me to lose my hair. Once it's lost I might as well complete the treatments.*

*They probably already have my chemo bags ready and they would be wasted if I didn't come out of the restroom.*

*Kristy and I could go shopping instead. We would have the whole afternoon to ourselves and that would give me more time to think.*

I suddenly realized I was being ridiculous. I had to get back to the room or they would be coming after me. As much as I wanted to go home, there was no escaping, so I washed my hands and returned to my chair.

As soon as I situated myself in the recliner, one of the nurses brought a name tag which I used for the duration of my treatments. She offered me something to drink or eat. I decided on a cold apple juice which she set on the table next to my recliner. Pulling over a handy machine on wheels, she took my temperature and blood pressure. I hung on to one last hope that my blood pressure would be too high to start today's treatment. Unfortunately, everything looked great. Next, the nurse brought over the materials needed to start an IV. The sound of the sterile instruments being released from their wrappers caused a knot to form in my stomach. (I still associate that sound with sharp instruments and pain.)

Oncology nurses are experts at starting IVs. I was really impressed with the skill my nurse used in quickly preparing me to be hooked up to the machine next to my chair. After successfully inserting the IV needle and taping it in place, she brought a pillow so my arm would be comfortable.

I came to know and love the nurses in the chemo room. Every nurse I met was genuinely caring, positive, and cheerful. I liked being around each of them and it was obvious they loved helping people through a difficult experience. Besides performing the important job of making sure all the patients were receiving the correct medicine and handling it well, they also gave us much needed comfort and support. They smiled, and that made all the difference.

The room was pretty full that day, but I remember a woman about my age enter the room not more than ten minutes after me. I probably noticed her because she looked like I felt. I chuckled inside when I heard a nurse tell her, "We already had another patient try to get out of having chemo by escaping to the restroom and telling us she was too tired. You don't have to be rested to receive chemo!" At least I wasn't the only one going through chemo anxiety.

With tubes connecting me to the IV pole, I was committed. What words can adequately explain how it feels to finally acquiesce to something that will be good for you, but at the same time bad for you?

The first few bags they brought were pre-meds. I didn't ask many questions this first day, but I did figure out that one bag prevented nausea. After about fifteen minutes, the preliminary bags had emptied and a nurse brought a bulging bag filled with clear liquid. By the end of the day I figured out it was the "C" of the "TAC" package because "A" was forced into my IV using a syringe and "T" was given last.

Once the larger bag was positioned on my pole and connected to my IV, Kristy and I played the card game I brought. When we tired of that, we just visited. I kept my eye on all that was going on around me, watching the nurses attend to other patients. The room was generally quiet with little movement except for nurses changing bags when the machines beeped to signal it was time, or the occasional patient exiting to use the restroom. With so much liquid dripping into our veins, it was typical to make a few trips during the three to four hours of infusion. I learned from observation this was accomplished by unplugging the machine and dragging the pole, bags and all, with me. It was a little awkward, but manageable.

As I glanced around, the thought came to me that each person in that chemo room had a story. They weren't just people with cancer, but unique individuals with feelings, hopes, and dreams. We were all sitting solemnly, trusting in our doctors and hoping that the strong drugs we were allowing to invade our bodies would be enough to overpower the enemy.

As the first large bag emptied, announced by the repetitive beeping of my machine, the nurse returned to begin the next drug. I learned that this one was often referred to by chemo patients as the "Red Devil". It was the culprit that caused hair to fall out and instead of being administered from a bag, it came in two really fat syringes. True to its nickname, it was Kool Aid red.

The nurse attached the syringe to my IV, slowly pushing the red liquid into my veins. There was something eerie about this drug. First, I was receiving it forcefully from a syringe, and secondly I knew it would be causing hair loss in ten to fourteen days. As I watched the first syringe empty, knowing that the contents were coursing through my bloodstream, I wondered where the strength was coming to allow this. It's one thing to have a bag hanging from a pole that you can ignore, and another to visibly observe the drug being administered. I reached a point where I couldn't watch anymore and started a meaningless conversation with Kristy. Again, I felt the loss of control. I succumbed, but not without trepidation.

Having completed this phase of my treatment, I faced one more bag, which like the first, would drip through the IV. It was the "T" of my TAC cocktail, and I was relieved to be almost done for the day. My friend Lauri had made me a chemo chart, providing stickers to mark the completion of each treatment. When I went home, I could place the first sticker on the chart and rejoice in having just five remaining sessions.

As the nurse placed the final bag on the hook and plugged it into my IV, I sat back, anxious to be finished and free to go home. I felt like I had been in that chemo room for such a long time, and I was cold. It was a different kind of chill, the kind that sank into your bones. I snuggled under the fleece blanket I had brought and continued to visit with my daughter.

I was about ten minutes into this final chemo treatment when suddenly my chest tightened and I found it difficult to breathe. It happened so quickly; a normal breath out followed by a labored attempt to draw one in. I whispered to Kristy,

"Tell the nurses I can't breathe."

Kristy quickly jumped up and ran over to the nurses' desk to relay my message and the room suddenly became animated. One nurse turned off the machine pumping the Taxotere into my veins. Before I knew it, another machine with an oxygen mask was wheeled in front of me, and Dr. Polowy was listening to my chest with his stethoscope. I wondered where he came from as I never saw him walk into the room. A nurse was taking my vitals while he listened, and within a matter of minutes, I could breathe normally again. This was undoubtedly due to the fact the drug was no longer entering my body.

The doctor looked relieved and spoke for a few minutes with a nurse and left. I was told they were going to try the Taxotere again, but not before giving me some antihistamines. When they did resume the Taxotere drip, it would be administered slowly. I wasn't exactly thrilled they were still planning on giving me this last drug, but I had to trust their judgment. I was on edge until the machine announced the bag had emptied.

Due to the additional allergy meds administered, and the slow dripping of the Taxotere, my first chemo session exceeded four hours. With the interventions, I was able to tolerate the full dose of the last drug, but I was truly worn out when I arrived home. I fell into the comfort of my bed, not even bothering to put the first sticker on my chemo chart. The excitement I had anticipated over having a session completed was wiped out by extreme physical exhaustion I could not have imagined.

Since I didn't sleep well the night before, I spent the afternoon in bed sleeping off and on. Friends brought us dinner which I didn't feel like eating, but at least my family could make good use of it. I wasn't nauseated, simply too exhausted to care about food. It was the last evening Kristy would be with me, so I visited with her and read a story to my grandson. I would miss their company and help, but was later grateful they didn't have to witness the following days when everything went drastically downhill.

The next day, Randy drove me back to the Cancer Center to receive my Neulasta shot. The purpose of this injection was to build up the white blood cells destroyed by the chemo. When the nurse entered the injection room, she asked if I wanted to receive the shot in my arm or stomach. I asked what most people chose and she replied the stomach, a less painful approach. Getting a shot in the stomach didn't sound appealing to me, but I took her word for it and opted for the fleshier area of my abdomen. The nurse was a master at administering this shot and I experienced little pain. Unlike the day before, my visit was brief and I was grateful to soon be on my way.

I wished I was going home, but instead, I had an appointment at the imaging center to get an ultrasound of my thyroid. Apparently, a spot showed up on the PET scan and the doctor wanted a closer look. When the nurse called with this report, I numbly received it, resigning myself to the fact that the drama was not over. I was beginning to feel there was never going to be an end to the bad news concerning my health. Was cancer silently invading other areas? How was it possible for it to be so sneaky, slithering wherever it wanted, choosing any available spot to multiply and grow? As I lay on the table feeling the ultrasound probe move over my gelled neck, I gave myself a pep talk to keep the tears from forming.

As each day went by after my first chemo, I felt increasingly worse. I received my treatment on Wednesday and true to prediction, I had reached a low point on Saturday and Sunday. I managed my nausea by taking the prescribed medicine every four hours, before it reached the point of being out of control. I tried to drink plenty of liquids, which was not easy for me. The oncology nurses, along with instructions in the chemo notebook, stressed the importance of drinking 64 ounces of liquid per day. Plain water brought on nausea so I tried flavored waters and Gatorade. I couldn't tolerate cold liquids, so I drank them at room temperature. Trying my best, I was only able to get down a little more than half of each day's requirement. The worse I felt, the less I was able to drink.

Eating presented additional concerns for my husband as he visibly noted my declining energy. When I needed to be gaining strength from food, my appetite waned. It was similar to how I felt the first trimester of my pregnancies. If something sounded appealing, it shifted to disgusting by the time it was prepared. Randy tried to tease my appetite by offering my favorite foods.

"How about some shrimp or salmon tacos? I'll run and get some for you."

"No thanks. That doesn't sound good right now." Under normal conditions, I never turn down Mexican food. Randy says I should have been born Latino.

He was confident I wouldn't pass up his next offer. "I can bring you a bowl of mint chocolate chip ice cream!" I'm sure he was thinking that at least it was a dairy product. I normally love ice cream, especially mint chocolate chip. Unfortunately, my stomach wouldn't tolerate ice cream, or anything sweet, during all the months I received chemo.

"I can make you a scrambled egg sandwich."

"Now I'm really going to throw up." He knows I don't like eggs.

"Tuna sandwich?"

"Are you kidding?" Sadly, my husband doesn't have a very long list of things he is comfortable making.

"What about grilled cheese?"

"Ok. I'll try that."

Looking at the nicely grilled sandwich Randy brought, I sighed, "Maybe a bowl of cereal would taste better."

After I choked down two bites of cereal, Randy, who never likes to waste food, reluctantly threw the rest out. I might sound a little spoiled here, but in reality, I had no interest in eating and what I did eat during my worst days after chemo was only due to the insistence of my patient husband.

I felt so tired, but not a sleepy kind of tired. It was an overwhelming fatigue that I've never experienced. To make matters worse, I couldn't sleep, day or night. My legs felt fidgety and the muscles wouldn't relax, causing me to want to pace the floor. Being too worn out to do so, I just lay in bed, moving my legs back and forth but receiving no relief from the restlessness. When I did drift off to sleep, it would be for short periods, waking to face more of the same. If I could best sum up how I felt, it would be a combination of being pregnant and having the flu at the same time.

What did I do during all the hours of lying in bed awake? I remembered back to a conversation I had with my friend Cindy when she was recovering from a chemo treatment.

"Look at all the time you have to read! How many books have you read since you started chemo?"

"None. I can't concentrate enough to read anything. I just lay here." I couldn't believe it. I thought then how I would love to have a reason to lie around and read all the books I hadn't had a chance to open yet.

Now I understood. I had no desire to go to my bookshelf and choose one of the many volumes that called my name when I walked by. Once I attempted an easy-read fiction to divert my attention on how I was feeling. I never got past the first chapter.

It was the same with watching movies, which required even less mental effort or concentration. I simply was not interested, even when someone offered to start one for me. A movie was more annoying than entertaining. What a shame to have all this time and no yearning or energy to make use of it. Typically, my personality dictated filling every moment with productive activity. Fortunately, I didn't have enough oomph to feel guilty about my lack of accomplishment.

There was time to think. Plenty of time. Too much time. I thought about my second-grade class. *How was the new school year going?* My students didn't miss me because they didn't know me. I didn't miss them because right now they were blank faces. *Was Lori able to carry out my lesson plans? Were the students learning the classroom routines and expectations? How was I going to merge into what has been established?* I felt so estranged from my own classroom. I thought about the present. *When would Randy get home? What sounds good to eat? Why can't I sleep? Should I call Cindy? Later. I don't feel like talking. Should I get up and go to the bathroom? Later. I'm too tired to move.*

I was scheduled to return to school on Wednesday of the following week, seven days after my first treatment. On Monday morning I wasn't feeling better, but I still had to make a trip to the lab for my weekly blood work. A friend took me as I didn't feel strong enough to drive myself the short three miles. The trip completely wore me out and I returned to bed for another day of feeling miserable. I had developed a bad case of diarrhea which added to my discomfort and forced me out of bed more than I wanted.

On Monday evening, I changed locations from my bed to the couch and tried to watch a little TV with Randy. The only thing I felt like eating was oatmeal. As I finished it, I felt worse than ever and walked to my bedroom. By the time I got there, I broke out in a cold sweat and rushed into the bathroom, certain I was going to throw up. Brittany sat at the computer in my room, and not wishing to worry her, I tried to suppress the overwhelming urge to vomit. When the feeling finally passed, I walked towards my bed when a sudden burst of dizziness caused me to collapse. Luckily, I had reached the side of the bed in time or I would have fallen on the floor. Landing on my bed, I didn't move, hoping for the feeling to pass. Brittany looked up from her homework and ran to get her dad. When Randy arrived and saw how pale and listless I was, he helped me under the covers and tried to get me to drink some water. I agreed to the water if he also brought my nausea medicine. Placing both on my night stand I attempted to go to sleep, if only to escape how badly I was feeling.

As tired as I was, sleep didn't come easily. I was aware that chemotherapy could be difficult and I tried to patiently endure, but I was beginning to question my ability to go through this five more times. I wasn't even close to feeling good enough to teach school the day after tomorrow. Would it be possible to teach at all? Being sick was hard enough without the guilt I felt for not fulfilling my obligations.

Morning brought no relief from the weakness and sickness that wracked my body. It had been a long night with little sleep. I felt like I had a bad case of the flu. Randy brought more fluids and encouraged me to drink. He also brought me some toast for breakfast then reluctantly went to work. I looked deathly sick to him and if it weren't for patients depending on him to be there that day, he wouldn't have left. Years later he shared with me his frightening thought, "Cancer isn't going to kill her. Chemo is."

With Brittany in school, I was left alone to wait out the day, hoping to soon feel better. It took great effort to get out of bed and use the bathroom but the diarrhea necessitated frequent trips. I felt like someone had zapped all the energy out of my body and I no longer agonized over my inability to teach school the next day. I didn't care about anything.

About mid-morning, my cell phone rang. The caller ID showed "Private Call" and I almost didn't answer it. It was a good thing I did because it was Dr. Dinsdale, my primary care doctor. In a concerned voice, he explained that the results of the previous day's blood work had been mistakenly sent to his office and it didn't look good. He needed to know my oncologist's name so he could fax it over for his attention. Despite the Neulasta shot I had received, my white blood cell count was "0".

"How are the fluids? Are you drinking plenty of water?"

"I'm trying to," I answered feebly, "but drinking makes me nauseated."

"About how much have you kept down this morning."

"Maybe four ounces."

"Claudia, that is not enough. You will end up in the hospital if you don't increase your fluid intake."

Right then I didn't even care. All I wanted to do was lay there and be left alone.

Within the hour, a nurse from my oncology office called. She explained that I needed to come in that day for a Neupogen shot to build up my white blood cells. I was to also plan on receiving this shot for two additional days. I told her I didn't feel like coming in. She firmly made it clear I had no choice, the Neupogen shot was essential, and they would see me at three o'clock.

As I hung up from this conversation, I wondered how in the world I was going to get out of bed and make the trip to the oncology office. I obviously couldn't drive myself, but with one call I found Monica willing to drop everything and take me. Until it was time to leave I just lay in bed, trying to obediently drink as much as possible. My doctor's warning had finally concerned me and I didn't want to be hospitalized. That would require too much energy.

About five minutes before Monica was to arrive, I dragged myself out of bed and got dressed. I ran a comb through my hair and brushed my teeth. I never leave the house without a shower and make-up but for once I didn't even care. I just wanted to get the shot and return to my bed.

When I arrived at the office, I was immediately taken to the injection room. It was a relief to get right to the reason for my visit. I couldn't wait to go back home, although I didn't feel much better there. I had barely sat down in the chair when two nurses came in to evaluate my situation. After asking a few questions, one administered the shot and the other left the room, only to return to announce that Dr. Polowy had ordered hydration. She explained, "You are extremely dehydrated and this will not only help alleviate the situation, but assist you in feeling better."

I was taken to the chemo room and given another IV which was hooked up to a large bag of clear liquid. Thinking of Monica who was only planning on bringing me for a shot I asked, "How long is this going to take?"

"It'll take about two hours. Do you have someone waiting for you?"

"Yes. My friend brought me. Would you mind bringing her in to be with me?"

"Not at all. I'll be right back."

Luckily, Monica was fine with the unexpected delay. I didn't feel like talking, but just reclined in the chair and stared at all that was happening around me. At one point, a nurse came over and asked if I was still having diarrhea, which I confirmed. She returned later with a prescription for this problem and a lab slip. I was to bring a sample of my stool tomorrow to rule out some malady I don't remember. When the hydration bag finally emptied, I escaped to use the restroom.

As I came out of the restroom, I nearly bumped into Dr. Polowy who was waiting for me. It was at this moment that I discovered the depth of compassion my oncologist possessed. I was moved by the look of concern in his eyes for the adverse reaction to my first round of chemo. He invited me to sit down in the injection room and positioned himself on a rolling stool next to me so we could converse face to face.

"I want you to come in every day this week to receive hydration. You'll be receiving two more Neupogen shots to raise your white cell count."

I remembered reading in my chemo handbook about possible reactions to Neupogen. "Isn't that the one that causes flu-like symptoms? I already feel like I have the flu."

"It might." I appreciated his honesty. "I've given you a prescription for the diarrhea. It's important we get that under control. Are you having any other discomforts?"

I mentioned my throat hurt and after looking at it, he wrote another prescription for an antibiotic. Remembering my thyroid ultra sound, I asked if he had received the results yet.

A look of concern crossed his face. "We will need to have the thyroid biopsied at some point. Right now, it is enough to focus on the breast cancer. We'll deal with the thyroid later."

Well that was a lovely piece of news. On top of everything, I could have thyroid cancer as well.

Being sensitive to my look of defeat, he brought the subject back to the present situation. "Every treatment doesn't have to be this bad. When you come in for your next appointment, we'll discuss some alternatives. I don't want you teaching school the rest of this week. You need to take care of yourself."

As he got up to leave the room, he turned, flashing me a smile of encouragement and simply said, "Hang in there."

I was never so glad to be back home in bed. This lengthy, unexpected trip to the doctor wore me out even further and I was not only sick, but exhausted. I obediently returned each day that week for an additional shot and further hydration. On one of those days, a nurse tried to get a blood sample from my IV for the lab. My veins weren't cooperating and she twisted the needle and moved it around until she received what she thought was enough to test my electrolytes. The experience wasn't pleasant, but I realized I had to get use to such procedures and learn to endure with more courage.

As each day passed, I began to feel better and my trips to the Cancer Center to receive hydration became tolerable. I passed the time by watching the patients in the infusion room. Some were not feeling well and sat quietly, or slept. Others joked with the nurses and visited with other patients. As the week went on, I found myself feeling well enough to converse with those around me as we shared our stories. I remember a young girl, probably in her twenties, who had brain cancer. How I ached to see her tread such a difficult path before she had experienced much of life. One very old man looked at me and said, "Was this your first chemo?" When I answered in the affirmative, he smiled and said, "The first one is always the worst."

On Friday, Dr. Polowy's nurse came in to check on me during my hydration. The lab report on my stool sample had come back negative but they were concerned that the medicine that had been prescribed on Tuesday hadn't taken care of the diarrhea.

"Dr. Polowy has prescribed opium as a last resort to combat the diarrhea. We have to get this under control."

I wasn't sure I heard her correctly. "He wants me to take WHAT?"

"Opium. It comes in a liquid form. An entire bottle costs around $400.00 but we're giving you a fourth of a bottle to begin with. Only one pharmacy carries this, which is luckily located in Mesa so you shouldn't have to go far to get it."

As I assimilated this new bit of information, she continued, "Dr. Polowy has ordered Home Health Care to come and administer hydration throughout the weekend. They'll come on both Saturday and Sunday."

She handed me some papers to fill out. I was grateful to have Randy with me. It was a lot to take in and even though I was feeling better than earlier that week, it didn't take much to deplete my small reserves of energy. I found some comfort in realizing I had successfully survived my first round of chemo, but it made me weary to think I still had five more to go.

The weekend brought a nurse to my home to administer yet another hydration. As she parked and wheeled in the IV pole, I hoped that none of my neighbors were watching. I didn't want any of my friends unnecessarily worrying. After filling out what I felt was my life history and signing multiple papers, the nurse was ready to start my IV.

She began by telling me it had been awhile since she had inserted an IV, information that I wished she hadn't disclosed. It's not a good idea to apologize before beginning a medical procedure. This confession probably didn't need to be shared because as she made the attempt, it was obvious she was a novice. She inserted the needle in a vein on top of my right hand. The vein rolled, causing her first attempt to be unsuccessful. She wasn't about to give up, trying several more stabs. By the time the task was accomplished, my hand was throbbing. It didn't stop hurting the entire two hours. As I sat there, I wondered if I should mention this, but decided against it since I didn't want her to take it out and try again. From this experience, I knew to never take for granted the oncology nurses who were experts at inserting an IV quickly and painlessly. Once the nurse could see all was running smoothly, she asked if she could leave to get some lunch. It was fine with me. I didn't want to entertain her for two hours.

When my hydration was complete, the nurse unhooked everything but left the IV needle in my hand, suggesting it could probably be used again the next day. She taped it down tightly so it wouldn't move. I wasn't sure if this was such a good idea because my hand was still throbbing from her many attempts to insert it earlier. I weighed the pros and cons of the matter, finally settling on keeping it in since who knew what tomorrow may bring.

The next day brought a different nurse and my final day of hydration. Skeptically, she looked at the needle in my hand and muttered, "I'm going to have to re-insert this IV. It looks like it's ready to fall out."

I had babied that needle all night, as well as endured the constant throbbing and was devastated at the thought of starting again. "Please. At least try and see if it will work," I pleaded.

She consented to try and mercifully it functioned to her satisfaction. I sustained a bruise for several weeks on the back of my hand as a little souvenir of my last two days of hydration.

The other memorable experience of that second weekend following my first chemo was taking the opium Dr. Polowy had prescribed as a final effort in eliminating the diarrhea. It came in a dark brown bottle with a dropper. The directions said to take one fourth of a dropper orally, four times a day. As soon as I opened the bottle, I knew I had a problem. The smell escaping it made me stagger backwards. How was I ever going to swallow it and keep it down? I found it really interesting that my family couldn't smell anything when I asked them to sniff the bottled contents. I had heard that an enhanced sense of smell was a possible side effect of chemo and this was proof.

I made the following preparations before each dose:
    Peel one third of a banana

> Pour a glass of milk
> Measure out one fourth dropper of opium
> Lay all of the above on a paper towel

Taking a deep breath, I would squeeze the opium into the back of my mouth, shove in the banana, chew a few times, and wash it all down with milk. I tried to do this without breathing so I wouldn't taste anything, but a residual taste remained. Luckily, I could keep it down. Even more fortunate was that it worked and I only had to take it for two days. Worse than the taste was the constant loopy feeling that came from this drug. Planning to teach school the next day, I was hoping to be free of the side effects of opium.

I had survived my first chemo treatment with Dr. Polowy's quick interventions. I wondered what he meant when he said he would modify my plan so I wouldn't suffer as much with subsequent treatments. I would just have to be patient until my next appointment to learn what was ahead.

By Monday, I was finally allowed to begin teaching school. It was like the first day of school for all of us. I was a stranger in my own classroom. Lori had managed well but now my little second-graders needed to adjust to me as their teacher.

I had learned a lesson from the previous week. Missing more days of school than I had previously planned placed Lori in a difficult situation. Since I had only submitted lesson plans through Tuesday, Lori, with the help of the other second-grade teachers, had to scramble to make it through the rest of the week. I felt bad and vowed from that point on to prepare more lessons in advance for the likely event of the unexpected happening.

Coming back was not easy. I was in a weakened condition, but had to use an excessive amount of energy to win my students' trust and respect. I also had to teach them the additional routines they needed to know for reading rotations as well as enforce my expectations. Since my typical beginning-of-the-year management practices hadn't been completely established yet, teaching was exhausting and I barely made it through the first week. In addition to teaching, I was spending time after school and on weekends to prepare lessons for the following two weeks. I wanted to be covered in case of the unknown, but this process was physically taxing.

During the ongoing months, I repeated this routine, consisting of a cycle of chemo treatments, recovery, catching up, and preparation, just so I could do it all over again. It was my mode of survival and it took all my energy, leaving no time for anything else. I was determined I could do anything for a few short months, as long as the end was still within reach.

*September 28, 2009*

*Dear Journal,*

*I just got home from the hospital after having my port placed. Lying on the bed next to me is the bright yellow, funny-shaped cap I wore during my surgery. It is evidence of an act of true charity performed on my behalf. Despite the difficult road I am asked to travel, there are moments that cause me to pause and wonder at the incredible goodness I find in the people I meet along the way. Sad to think I would've missed all this if my life had remained on an easy course.*

5

# THE NEW PLAN

Since my last recovery from chemo had taken longer than expected, it was time for my second treatment before I knew it. I only had eight days with my students. They were slowly adjusting and we were developing the necessary bond between teacher and student. I was reluctant to leave them before this was accomplished.

My appointment was scheduled for 2:30 p.m. on Wednesday and I decided this time I would return to school on Thursday. Judging from my last experience, I was basically tired on Thursday and Friday, so maybe I could miss less school by trying to teach those two days before I began feeling my worst. I hadn't considered the fact that my white blood cell count would be at its lowest and I would be subjecting myself to a myriad of germs that often accompany a classroom full of children.

Monica drove me to my appointment and this time I walked into the waiting room with more confidence. I had gone through these doors several times now since my introductory appointment with Dr. Polowy. The office wasn't foreign to me anymore, and although I wasn't entirely comfortable with it, at least I was familiar with the procedures. Becoming comfy with a cancer center is not on most peoples' bucket lists.

I walked over to the desk to sign my name on a sheet attached to a clipboard and checked the appropriate boxes stating if there were any recent labs drawn or scans performed. I sat down until the receptionist called my name, only to return to sign a yellow paper that indicated what was being done that day for insurance purposes. Unlike my previous visits, however, the receptionist asked to see my picture ID. I retrieved it for her, thinking how silly it was to have to show identification and I couldn't help but remark, "So, do you have many people come in and pretend they are someone else so they can have chemo?"

The receptionist smiled at my flimsy attempt at a joke, but didn't say a word. Of course, it was just a matter of procedure. She made a copy of it and never asked to see it again.

As I waited to see Dr. Polowy, I reviewed my little notebook of questions. This was my second appointment with him and I knew it would be different from the first when I learned about my cancer and his plan to eliminate it. I was anxious to hear how he was going to make my subsequent chemo treatments more tolerable. I had already lost my hair and was wearing a wig. It chose to fall out exactly thirteen days after my first treatment, only two days after entering my classroom to teach for the first time that year. Jumping into teaching after losing my hair, still weak from surgery and chemo, took strength that I had to dig deep to find. (Losing my hair was a traumatic event, even though I expected it. Chapter 6 is entirely devoted to the details of this experience.)

As I reflected on the past three weeks since my first chemo, I marveled at all that had transpired. My first treatment was anything but pleasant and I wasn't anxious for a repeat performance. When I was finally strong enough to teach, I was a stranger to my students. They had naturally adapted to my substitute and my sudden appearance was more of an interruption than a welcome. Lori had done an excellent job, but adjustments had to be made and it wasn't smooth.

My energy of previous years was absent and I struggled each day to provide for my students what they deserved, and manage their behavior. Where did the strength come to get through those first weeks? I honestly can't tell you. I plodded forward, unable to change anything, succumbing to my new life. I found if I wore a smile, people would assume all was well and not ask me questions I couldn't answer.

I clearly remember the first day back when the students were sitting on the big throw rug where we gather for calendar or stories. I looked into a sea of faces and realized I could only call about ten of them by name. When they were at their desks with name tags it was easy, but now they were shuffled out of order on the floor. A teacher is at a great disadvantage until she learns each child's name and I knew I had to quickly resolve this problem. When they returned to their desks, I concentrated on putting a name with a face. There were two little blond girls that looked very similar and for weeks I confused one for the other. Lacking continuity in my attendance didn't make the task of getting to know my students an easy one.

I was jolted back to the present when my name was called. I went through the same procedures as my previous appointment with the nurse recording my weight and leading me to an empty exam room. After taking my temperature and blood pressure, I was left to wait for my oncologist. I tried to imagine how Dr. Polowy would be changing my treatment plan. I was thankful for a doctor who paid attention to what I had gone through and was willing to adapt to my needs.

Dr. Polowy entered the room with a smile. First, he showed me the results of my recent blood work on his lap top. I stared at the screen, not sure what to focus on, but listened intently as he spoke. My white blood count had risen and all looked great to proceed with my chemotherapy today.

He apologized for the lousy experience I had with my first treatment, then explained the two options that would help prevent such severe side effects. He could either reduce the doses of my chemo drugs, or he could split them, giving me five more treatments of AC together, followed by five additional treatments of Taxotere.

Before I could comment, he quickly shared his opinion on which option was best. He wasn't in favor of lowering the dosage and recommended that we split the treatments as well as change from three-week to two-week intervals. Today I would only receive the AC combination.

I really liked the idea of coming every two weeks, which would help soften the blow of lengthening the time I would be receiving chemo. My mind quickly calculated that instead of five remaining sessions, I would have ten chemo treatments at two week intervals equaling a total of twenty weeks, or roughly five months. My end date would be extended, but by only a few weeks.

Continuing, Dr. Polowy recommended that I have a port placed which would make it easier on my veins with the additional treatments and the weekly requirement for blood samples. Since I had already observed others in the infusion room receive their chemo through a port, I was familiar with the device. From what I could see, it was round, about the size of a nickel, and protruded only slightly from under the skin. Placing a port could be accomplished by my surgeon, Dr. Deyden. After what I went through with the home health nurse, I could see the benefits.

I felt my discussion with Dr. Polowy was a good one and I entered the chemo room grateful that today's session would be shorter.

My decision to return to school on Thursday went well, although I was low on energy and patience. After school, I had to travel to the Cancer Center to receive my Neupogen shot. All that activity wore me out and as soon as I got home, I crawled in bed and stayed there all evening. I was still determined to make it through one more day, knowing that I would have the weekend to completely rest.

By noon on Friday I began fading quickly and I called Lori to come in and help. Being too tired to contribute, I sat all afternoon at my desk while Lori taught. That was the last time I attempted to attend school the two days after my treatment. Even though I wasn't violently sick, I was weak and void of energy.

Saturday and Sunday were my two worst days. I stayed in bed and tried to control the nausea with medicine and small, bland meals. I was relieved I didn't suffer extreme diarrhea like last time, and the flu-like symptoms were much milder. It looked like my oncologist's new plan was going to work.

On Monday, I developed a deep cough. I called the nurses' line that morning and was told to call back if I felt worse during the day. By late afternoon, my chest hurt and the cough worsened so I phoned the office and got the doctor on call. He prescribed an antibiotic and decongestant and within twenty-four hours I was feeling better. I was able to return to the classroom by Wednesday, when my white blood cell count had risen sufficiently and my infection was under control.

Returning to school the day after chemo was not a wise choice. I had made that decision on my own, never informing my medical team. Forgetting that chemotherapy destroys the immune system, I voluntarily exposed myself to a classroom of children.

To help avoid further infections, Dr. Polowy advised me to call each week to get the results of my blood work, informing me of the number my white blood cell count needed to reach before going out in public. This took the guess work out of when I could safely return to school.

The nurses also encouraged me to wear a mask when I taught, a suggestion I didn't embrace. It would be difficult to teach young children with my mouth covered, not to mention inhaling my own stuffy air all day. In addition, I was trying to avoid the appearance of looking sick, which was impossible while wearing a mask. Having a little too much pride, I risked the likelihood of exposing myself to the germs that were so prevalent during the Fall and Winter months.

Dr. Polowy decided to increase the number of Neupogen shots after this chemo, hoping that seven doses would sufficiently build up my white blood cell count in time for my next treatment in two weeks. I asked if my friend Monica could administer the shots, saving me daily trips, but when I called the pharmacy I found it would actually save money to go to my oncology clinic. To order the Neupogen serum would cost fifty dollars a shot and I would need seven after every chemo treatment. I was shocked at the price until the pharmacist told me this drug was costing my insurance company $800 per shot. Doing the math, I realized my insurance would be charged $5,600 for the seven injections following each AC treatment. It amazed me that anything could be that expensive and again I was thankful for good health insurance. I didn't even want to know what the chemo drugs cost.

Since the oncology clinic was closed on weekends, the office arranged for me to go to the hospital outpatient clinic to receive the necessary Neupogen shots. A day could not be skipped. The same two nurses were always there and I became friends with them. I enjoyed their cheerful attitudes and the care they gave. They were the best at giving the shot which had to be administered slowly in the stomach to prevent an uncomfortable burning. I always appreciated their gentle touch and sunny countenances, especially when it was the last place I wanted to go on the weekend, the two days I felt my worst.

I was now on a two-week schedule for receiving chemo, so it wasn't long before I was to return for my third treatment. I could tell I was feeling better mentally and physically because I decided to post all of my future treatments on a calendar, providing visual assurance that all of this would end. I also wanted to plan chemo around parent/teacher conferences as well as holidays such as Thanksgiving and Christmas. With calendar in hand, I was elated at my ability to reshape this portion of my crumbling world and regain a smidgen of control.

As I sat with Dr. Polowy I proudly pulled out my well-organized calendar and showed him my plan. He patiently listened but then presented me with the results of my blood work. My white blood cells were not recovering quickly enough to have chemo every two weeks and we would have to change our plan to a three-week rotation.

Was I hearing correctly? My attempt to chart the remainder of my chemo life was just shredded with one sentence. It didn't take a calculator to figure out that having to wait three weeks between treatments would push my ending date clear into Spring. My white cells hadn't even cooperated enough for me to have chemo today.

Dr. Polowy could sense my disappointment and tried to ease it by saying, "You are really normal. More people than you think are on a three-week cycle and have to split the chemo drugs. During our extra week, we'll have Dr. Deyden place your port and you'll be ready for the third treatment next Wednesday."

He went on to gently explain that I couldn't map my whole schedule of chemotherapy on a calendar because if I became sick or my blood count hadn't sufficiently risen, treatments would be delayed. We would just take it one treatment at a time. We could avoid personal conflicts, though, by moving my appointments back or ahead a few days. For example, on the week of parent/teacher conferences, I could have chemo at the end of the day on Friday instead of the middle of the week, allowing me to complete my responsibilities. I could see he was trying to help me understand the bitter fact that I couldn't plan chemo around my life. I needed to plan my life around chemo. As I sat facing my doctor in the exam room, the reality of that thought hit hard. I folded the pages of my calendar and slipped them in my purse, out of sight.

Giving in to this concept was far from easy for me. I felt defeated and incredibly discouraged about having to lengthen the amount of time I would be receiving chemotherapy. When I thought it was going to be six treatments, with one every three weeks, I had an ending date. When it changed to ten remaining treatments with each one administered every two weeks, I picked myself up and calculated a new date which was only about one and a half months later than the first. I could do that. Changing back to every three weeks with ten treatments to go was more than I cared to calculate. This was going to drag on much longer than I had planned.

To protect myself from further disappointment, I refused to estimate an ending date for the third time. If people asked when I would be finished with my treatments, I'd shrug my shoulders and reply, "I don't know." It wasn't until after Christmas when my school district wanted to know a tentative ending date that I finally counted the weeks on the calendar and told them the end of March or first of April.

I met with Dr. Deyden next to discuss the placement of a port. Randy was working so I went by myself. During this visit, Dr. Deyden explained what would take place and the risks involved. I didn't remember him giving me a list of risks before my mastectomy, which was major surgery, so I was somewhat shocked. He explained that I would be positioned completely flat on the operating table. Puncturing the lung was a possible risk since he would be working within a half inch of that organ. If my lung was punctured, I would experience a great deal of pain when the anesthesia wore off.

He also explained the risk factors after the port was placed, including infection or the port malfunctioning. If any microorganisms got in, they could go straight to my heart, causing major concerns. When he finished, I was seriously thinking of cancelling this out-patient surgery. The thought of my right arm's veins being depleted over the next eight months and the possibility of repeating the home nurse debacle presented a worse scenario, so I decided to take my doctor's advice and get the port.

The date was set for the following Monday. Unfortunately, the time was in the afternoon so I would have to fast all day. The fact that my white blood cell count was low didn't seem to bother either of my doctors and so I prepared in the areas I could. I called Lori to see if she could teach my class on Monday, and possibly Tuesday since I didn't know how I would react to the procedure. I had previously told Randy that he didn't need to cancel his patients and go with me since placing a port was such a simple matter, but after talking to Dr. Deyden, I was quietly regretting he wouldn't be there.

Even though it was an out-patient procedure, anesthesia would be required, prohibiting me from driving. Lauri was available and willing to take me, wait through the surgery, and accompany me home. That posed another problem, however. By this time, I had lost my hair. I recalled that the hospital provided a lovely blue paper cap to wear on the head during surgery, but I knew from experience it was magically gone upon waking in the recovery room. I was sensitive about people seeing me bald, especially my close friend. Everyone knew I was bald, but so far no one had a visual of my condition and quite frankly, I wanted to keep it that way. With more important worries surrounding me, it's strange that the image of my naked head lying on the hospital pillow for all to see bothered me so much.

On the day of surgery, I checked into the hospital at one o'clock. Like a few months before, I was shown a bathroom where I could change into a hospital gown, a paper cap and large slippers. As I removed my wig and placed the cap on, I was horrified to see that it was more transparent than I remembered and my bald head was clearly visible. There was nothing I could do about it so I walked to the waiting cubical and laid down on the hard bed, hoping everyone would overlook my oddly shaped hairless head. No one gets a port unless they are a cancer patient, so I don't know why I was so self-conscious. It wasn't as if I could hide my condition and pretend normality.

Lauri and I visited until the anesthesiologist came in and introduced herself. When she asked if I had any questions, I told her I didn't but I did have one request.

"When I wake up, I want this cap to still be on my head." Even though it didn't completely shield the eye from my shiny scalp, at least it masked it to some degree.

She understood what I meant and told me she would be right back. Returning, she brought a hospital cap made of bright yellow printed material. Volunteers had lovingly sewn such caps for youth cancer patients. It fit perfectly and completely hid my baldness. Her small act of kindness and compassion for my feelings helped me relax and I said a silent prayer of gratitude as they wheeled me into the operating room. I was only briefly aware of the cold and sterile surroundings before I was out.

Where does time go when you're under anesthesia? Moments of your life are completely lost. Each experience is essentially the same. There isn't even a dream to recall.

This time was no different. One minute I was alert, and somewhat apprehensive, and a split second later, I was barely awake in a strange room with people I'd never seen. Knowing the surgery was over, I felt a sense of relief and all I wanted to do was drift back to sleep. I was vaguely aware of the nurse telling me they were going to do an X-ray of my chest, to assure the port was placed correctly. Feeling no pain, I quickly drifted back to sleep, never remembering the X-ray.

The next thing I remember was Lauri sitting beside my bed and a nurse talking rapidly, giving instructions, as if I was fully awake. When the nurse left, Lauri smiled and briefly summarized the important points. Apparently, everything had gone smoothly and Dr. Deyden had left a device in the port, making it immediately accessible for my chemo treatment on Wednesday. I was grateful for that gesture since the area was tender and the last thing I wanted was a needle inserted into the reddened, tender skin.

After regaining some strength, it was time to get dressed and I was handed my bag of clothes. Lauri had been taking care of my wig in a separate bag so it wouldn't be tossed around, and I took them both and entered a nearby bathroom.

As I dressed, I looked in the mirror to get a glimpse of my new addition. It was completely covered with sterile gauze and tape except for the two-inch device that dangled free, providing easy access. At least now I could avoid the weekly pokes in my arm and hand. I was so thankful the placement of my port transpired smoothly and the procedure was over. I did wonder if my clothes would cover it as it seemed to have been placed rather high in my right upper chest area. The last thing I wanted was for anyone to see it.

The next day I drove to the oncology clinic to have blood drawn in preparation for Wednesday's chemo. Before leaving home, I decided to remove all the bandages surrounding the incision so the nurses could see what they were doing, a well-intentioned, but regrettable idea.

When I arrived, the nurse asked why I had removed the gauze dressing that was placed to protect the incision. I was surprised with the question and really didn't have an answer. I was disappointed to hear that now she couldn't use the device Dr. Deyden had placed since it was contaminated and she would have to remove it and access the port with a needle. I wasn't looking forward to another stick in a place that was still very sensitive and I wished I hadn't tampered with the bandages. Every time I tried to take matters into my own hands, I made a mess of things. I was gradually learning that my futile attempts to maintain some degree of control were not worth it.

On Wednesday, I returned to school to teach for the only day that week. After school was out, I would drive to my appointment with Dr. Polowy. Hopefully, my blood count had risen enough so we could proceed without further delay.

As Dr. Polowy entered the room, he cheerfully exclaimed, "Congratulations on your port!"

His remark amused me and I smiled thinking only a doctor would extend congratulations for a port. You never hear your friends extend best wishes on your brand-new port as they pass you on the street. "Hey! I heard you have a port! Where can I acquire such a fine apparatus?"

As he examined me, he remarked on what a superb job Dr. Deyden had done. "I'll have to call and tell him how good your port looks." How did I luck out in getting such an optimistic oncologist? He was definitely the bright spot in these dreaded chemo visits.

Dr. Polowy also cheerfully reported that my white blood cell count had barely risen enough to proceed with chemo. My treatment that day was uneventful and I was glad to have my third chemotherapy behind me.

One result of that day's appointment was Dr. Polowy's recommendation to increase my Neupogen shots following each chemo from seven to eight injections, hoping it would help bring my white cell count up to a higher level. I obediently went daily for these injections, driving to the Cancer Center immediately after school.

On the evening following my eighth shot I began having pains in my chest. It was a sensation I had never felt before, originating in my sternum and radiating outward. When I sat or lay down, it would worsen. I decided to take two Tylenol and go to bed, not mentioning the pain to Randy. I reasoned that I was probably overtired and needed to get some rest. I also took a sleeping pill since it was important I got a good rest to teach school the next day.

The sleeping pill helped me go to sleep immediately, but I kept waking up in a stupor following strange nightmares. Around 2:00 a.m., I finally came to my senses, realizing I was in a great deal of pain. My chest was hurting constantly. I grabbed my chemo notebook and went into another room and turned on the light. I scanned the pages of possible chemo side effects, even though it had been a full week since receiving my last treatment. I couldn't find anything that matched what I was experiencing. Could I be having a heart attack?

Walking around didn't help the pain, so I finally decided to wake Randy and get his advice about what I should do. He was worried, which didn't help me feel any better, and told me I needed to call my doctor.

Calling a physician in the middle of the night is on my list of ten least favorite things to do. I avoid it at all costs. When I protested, he urged me to do so anyway, but I couldn't decide which doctor to call. Should I call the oncology after-hours line, or my surgeon, Dr. Deyden? I finally decided on Dr. Deyden as it had only been a little over a week since my port was placed and perhaps the pain had to do with an infection. Upon reaching Dr. Deyden, and apologizing for waking him, he asked me a few questions and then suggested I go to the Emergency Room.

By then I was also experiencing the same kind of pain in my pelvis, which was confusing, but at least made me think it probably wasn't a heart attack. I quickly dressed and flopped on my wig, trudging reluctantly out to the car. It hurt to walk now and the pain in my chest increased.

Even though I'd made the trip to this very hospital many times in the last three months, it seemed longer in the wee hours of the morning. I wasn't looking forward to sitting in a waiting room for a long time and hoped this could be resolved quickly.

When we arrived, I was amazed at how active an Emergency Room can be at three o'clock in the morning. It was full of people coughing, children wrapped in blankets, and those that accompanied them pacing the floor. I was about fourth in line to check in and I tried desperately to keep my distance from the others.

When it was my turn, I explained my symptoms and asked if I could have a face mask as I was a cancer patient currently undergoing treatments. Upon hearing this, I was placed in a wheelchair and whisked to a private room away from the other patients. As much as I hated circumventing all those ahead of me, I was relieved to skip the waiting area and the possibility of being exposed to a myriad of ailments.

After changing into a gown, someone came in to perform an EKG. Immediately after that a nurse began an IV in my arm. I was given a choice of using my port, but decided against it since the incision was still healing and it could be the source of my problem. Blood was drawn and someone brought me warm blankets which provided some comfort.

This initial activity was followed by a long wait. At one point, I asked if I could take one of the nausea pills in my purse but instead they gave me medicine through my IV. Later a technician came in with an X-ray machine and took a picture of my chest. My nurse was very attentive and checked on me frequently to see if I was comfortable.

Since my first chemo, my treatments had not been kind. The unanticipated was what kicked me off balance. As soon as I thought I had the routine figured out and knew what to expect, something unusual would occur. I couldn't imagine what was causing my pain as it didn't fit any of the listed side effects in my chemo notebook. As I vented my frustration to Randy, he muttered, "I guess with cancer, you have to expect the unexpected."

This was my first experience with the Emergency Room. I had brought a family member before, a child, or my mom, but had never been a patient. I didn't like it here. Everyone that attended to me was kind enough, but it took a ridiculous amount of time for things to progress. I was stable, so I'm sure attention was given to those facing life-threatening situations.

At 6:00 a.m. I decided to call Brittany as I knew her alarm would be going off and she'd wonder why everyone in the house was gone. She didn't answer so I left a message, trying to sound cheerful and optimistic.

"Hi honey. This is Mom. Dad and I are at the hospital to check on some chest pains I had during the night. Everything seems to be going well and I should be home soon, but not before you have to leave for school. Everything is looking good, so don't worry. Just wanted you to know why we aren't home. Love you."

Later I learned how much this message upset her. She was already having difficulty dealing with cancer in our home, and now she woke up to the news that I was at the hospital. That day at school, she ended up in tears in the counselor's office. She was trying so hard to be strong, but being at school and not knowing what was going on was more than she could handle. Her counselor was familiar with the situation and was a great listener, assisting several times throughout the year in dealing with her constant worries. More than once I was grateful for those who stepped up to assist my youngest daughter, understanding that I was not the only one suffering.

Just like it is impossible for some to fully understand what a cancer patient goes through, I will never know to what extent Brittany suffered during the year I was diagnosed and treated for cancer. She tried to exercise her faith and appear positive, but cancer was taking its toll on her as well. It didn't help that her best friend's dad passed away from cancer just months before my diagnosis.

My mind flashed back to when Brittany was about four years old. I recalled times when she would ask, "Mom, are you going to get cancer?" I wondered where she came up with such a notion and replied, "Of course not." Not trusting my answer, she would make me promise I would never have cancer. Of course, I would appease her with promises that I felt were safe to give. I had forgotten about these unusual conversations until now. Perhaps she came to this earth with a premonition of what our family would ultimately face.

Next I called Lori to see if she could substitute for me as it didn't look like I would be getting out of the hospital in time to teach, even if I felt like it. Luckily, she was willing and ready. I called my school and left a message, asking the secretary if she would call and report my absence as I had left those numbers at home.

I had been in the Emergency Room for almost four hours and still hadn't seen a doctor. I couldn't help but think that my EKG and X-ray were normal or more would be happening. At times the pain would let up a little, making it almost possible to sleep, but sleep did not come.

As time ticked on, Randy asked if I wanted him to cancel his morning patients so he could continue to stay with me. I encouraged him to just go and get ready for work as I was stable and there wasn't much he could do. As he kissed me good-bye, tears unexpectedly streamed down my face. My sensible self didn't want him to miss work but it was hard to let go when we didn't have a clue what was going on.

At that point, the doctor walked in. What a relief it was to see him before Randy left. He reported that the results of the EKG and X-ray showed nothing amiss but he had ordered a CT scan to be certain they hadn't overlooked anything. He had also placed a call to Dr. Polowy to report my symptoms and get his input. It was a relief to finally talk to a doctor and hear all tests performed up to this point were normal. Having received an update, Randy felt comfortable about leaving and gave me another quick kiss before hurrying home.

My nurse returned shortly after the doctor left to give me morphine to help alleviate the pain. This was the first time I was given morphine; it worked quickly to help me relax, but only dulled the pain. I had never experienced chest pains like this before, which undoubtedly contributed to my anxiety. It was confusing to also have pelvic pain, being identical to what I felt in my chest. Surely the cause would be the same.

Left alone, I lay in the private room listening to occasional sirens and the constant activity outside. I wondered about others who had come for help that morning or were brought in by ambulances. I may have dozed, but if so, it was only for brief moments. I looked forward to having this matter resolved and going home to my own bed. I was getting hungry, but was only allowed ice chips.

I can't be sure how much time passed before someone came to take me for the CT scan. As they rolled the bed out of my enclosed room, I covered my face with the mask they provided, hoping to avoid germs from all the coughing patients waiting to be seen by the doctor. I couldn't afford to be sick outside of the expected recovery from each chemo treatment and being in the Emergency Room was like residing in a petri dish.

When we entered the room with the huge CT scan machine, I climbed onto the table that rolled under the camera. As luck would have it, the nurse was having a difficult time getting my IV to take the required dye and she muttered that she may need to start a new one. She finally got it to work and I breathed a sigh of relief. Since I had experienced a CT scan before, I was familiar with the warm sensation that coursed through my body as the dye was administered.

The CT scan completed, we returned to my isolated room in the E.R. There I waited until the doctor would get the results of my latest imaging and then find time to return and give me a report.

It was a lonely wait with Randy gone and I had plenty of time to think. So much had happened since that summer day in July when I learned I had cancer. I spent more time going to doctors, having my blood drawn, and being in bed during the last four months than my entire life up to that point. Most of the time I didn't feel good and I never slept well. I didn't enjoy participating in the things I use to love doing. Teaching school wasn't bringing me the joy it had in years past and I had a hard time getting into the routine each time I returned. Now, a middle of the night rush to the Emergency Room for chest pains. What would next week bring? Cancer was dreadfully unpredictable.

My ears perked up when I heard the loud speaker proclaim, "Dr. Polowy calling for Dr. Moss." Dr. Moss was my Emergency Room doctor and apparently, Dr. Polowy was returning his call about my condition. I was hoping that I would have some answers before long and be able to go home. Before the doctor walked in however, I was surprised to see Randy. He entered with a big smile on his face. One of his patients cancelled so he left his office to see how I was doing. What an enormous boost to my morale to see him again and I was hopeful he would be able to take me home before he had to return to work.

Around 11:00 a.m. Dr. Moss entered my room and sat down to share his findings. He first assured me that all the tests had come back with good results. My heart was fine as well as my lungs. He had spoken with Dr. Polowy and had given him a rundown of my symptoms and the tests performed. Dr. Polowy and Dr. Moss agreed on what was causing the pain in my chest and pelvis. I had received too much Neupogen. Dr. Moss went on to explain that white blood cells are produced in bone marrow which is found in several bones but concentrated mostly in the sternum and pelvis. Neupogen was stimulating my marrow to make more white blood cells, and this led to a side effect of bone pain. What felt more like a heart attack was just an unfortunate adverse event related to this immune booster. Dr. Polowy would have to cut back to seven Neupogen shots as the eighth shot proved to be one too many. Remedy? Go home and wait it out, taking pain medication until the drug wore off.

I was relieved to know my heart was fine and I was thankful the cause of my pain had been determined. I couldn't help but think that this rush to the Emergency Room might have been avoided if I had called the oncologist in the early morning hours instead of Dr. Deyden. Perhaps they would have recognized the symptoms, common to cancer patients, and suggested I take pain medication to see if that helped.

At any rate, I learned to recognize bone pain and not panic when I experienced it, which did reoccur several times during my chemo treatments, although not as severe as the first. Dr. Polowy had also learned my limitations on the drug. From that day on, I never received more than seven shots in a row. The adjustment still accomplished its purpose, although many times just bringing the count to barely above the minimum in time to receive my next chemo treatment.

Randy was able to remain with me until I was released from the hospital. On the way home, he decided to get us something for lunch and we stopped at a favorite sub sandwich restaurant. I was famished since it was now almost noon and I eagerly ate my meal. That was the last time I enjoyed that particular restaurant. For some reason, the smell of those subs triggered an unpleasant memory which has taken several years to erase.

Now that I was only receiving the drugs AC at each three-week visit, my reactions to each chemo treatment had lessened considerably. The medicine I had been given for nausea worked well as long as I took it regularly.

Probably the most annoying side effect was my inability to relax or sleep. I never napped during the day, although I was extremely tired from little sleep the night before. I would frequently get out of bed and pace the floor, even though I rarely felt like exerting the energy. I was constantly fidgety and found that reading or watching a movie didn't quiet the restlessness that racked my extremities. Brittany would often encourage me to watch a movie, but nothing she suggested sounded the least bit enticing. She hated seeing me just lie there, so she would put one on anyway, trying to help however she could.

During these times, I basically did nothing, looking forward to Randy's visits during his lunch break from work. His presence was calming and he would often fix or buy me lunch. Sometimes I would visit with family or friends on the phone, but even too much visiting wore me out. I learned to endure these long days and looked forward to the promise of better ones ahead.

Sometimes as these moments of anxiety and restlessness subsided, I would force myself to grade school papers. I always had a huge pile of second-grade work to check. On the days that I taught and prepared for my next absence, I never had enough energy to also do the grading, so I would throw it all into a pile to check while recovering from chemo. This routine worked relatively well, even though there were many times I would literally have to force myself to plow through the stack. My reward for the effort was getting to see how my students were doing. The problem, though, was never knowing who in my class was falling behind or didn't understand a concept until weeks had passed.

Saving papers to grade was definitely not the recommended route, but it was the only way I could get through the year. As with everything else lately, I would have to make the best of the situation and hope my students would not be negatively affected by my limitations. I was doing the best I could, but it never measured up to my high standards of performance. This was one of the hardest things I had to accept during these difficult, trying days.

*September 1, 2009*

*Dear Journal,*

*This evening my hair began to fall out. Mack responded immediately and met me at his salon, just blocks from my house. What could have been an evening of distress was rescued by Mack's sense of humor. In one hour, it was done.*

*As Randy held my hand and walked me to the car, it was sprinkling lightly, a relatively rare phenomenon in Arizona. Perhaps the heavens understood and were shedding a few tears for my loss.*

# HAIR TODAY, GONE TOMORROW

Chemo is hair's worst enemy. One of my greatest concerns about receiving chemo was losing my hair. Hair loss is the most visible side-effect of having cancer. It was something I couldn't shove into my cancer file to deal with later. When I began losing my hair, I discovered I was dealing with more than the hair on my head. It included my eyebrows and eyelashes, giving me a sallow, sickly look. On a positive note, it also took into account the hair on my legs and under my arms. I didn't need to shave during my entire chemo treatment.

Many women spend a great deal of time and money styling and maintaining their hair. I paid a considerable sum every month for a professional trim and color. To add to the cost of this upkeep, I always bought the expensive brands of shampoos and conditioners. Searching for the positive in my impending baldness, I calculated how much money I would save during the next year. It was a substantial amount and provided some consolation for the upcoming dreaded event.

In my quest to look on the bright side, I also realized I would not have to worry about "bad hair days". Remembering mornings when my hair decided to have a mind of its own, I knew I wouldn't miss those battles. Wind, rain, and humidity would no longer have a say in the day's styling outcome. After I lost my hair I saw bad hair days from a whole new perspective. What I would give to have hair, no matter how it looked.

I always loved the feel of hair on my face. I generally styled it to bring out a more feminine, softer look. I've never been a lover of really short hair, although most of my life I've worn it in a pixie style. Sometimes, for variety, I'd grow it longer but seldom past my shoulders. My features are small so short to medium hair always looked best. That was not to say that I didn't dream of having long, gorgeous hair, flowing down my back. Growing up, I equated long hair and curls with femininity, which might explain my dismay in having no hair.

I remember my hair being long when I was a little girl. My mom would often braid it after brushing it vigorously. I clearly recall standing in our bathroom while she brushed out my tangles. My hair was fine and thick and so the snarls were ever present. In my little girl mind, something that hurt must be tangible and so I'd insist on seeing the knots my mom worked so hard to brush out. I could never understand why she couldn't produce one for me to examine. The nasty tangles were probably what motivated her to cut my hair into a shorter style and there it remained for most of my youth.

In high school, I coveted long hair. At the time, long, straight hair was the rage. If you were one of the truly unfortunate ones born with natural curls, you ironed them straight. There was one girl in my English class who had the most gorgeous hair I had ever seen. It flowed past her waist and was completely straight and thick. It must have taken her years to get it to that length. At the time, my hair was short with many layers and so the likelihood of copying her was nil. By the time I got past all the awkward stages and to one length, my high school years would be over and the styles would change. It didn't keep me from wishing, though, and I was convinced I'd truly be beautiful if only my hair was long.

When I ended up being the mother to five daughters, they all had long, gorgeous hair which was a delight to me. I never tired of fixing their thick locks in everything from French braids to pony tails to curls which of course included bows and ribbons. I can't even describe the volume and variety of hair adornments five little girls can own. There was one entire bathroom cabinet devoted to their storage. All five daughters chose to keep their long hair through their teens, a tribute to what I had always longed to have.

When I learned I had cancer, my hair was between my chin and shoulders. It had taken several years to grow from a shorter, layered look to a bob, which I jazzed up with some highlights. I loved my current look and the thought of losing all my hair and starting from scratch made me sick.

I had a hard time imagining myself bald. The last time I was close to being bald was when I was born, and even then I had some hair. I could only hope I might escape this curse and be one of the lucky ones that the chemo did not affect. That's how little I knew about the drugs I would be given. No one escapes hair loss, at least with the chemo cocktail I would be assigned.

My surgeon had already affirmed that I would be losing my hair, but just to be sure I asked Dr. Polowy. I was hoping I would hear, "Maybe" or "Most likely," but instead I heard an unequivocal "Yes." It wasn't said with much sympathy either. From a doctor's point of view, the loss of hair is a minor inconvenience in saving a life, for which I would have to agree. The word "Yes" was quickly followed by, "But it will grow back." That was not much reassurance. At a speedy record of one half inch per month, it would be quite some time before my hair would return to its present length.

Have you noticed that when you are about to lose something and you know it, you begin to appreciate it more? I loved running my fingers through my hair, feeling its weight as I washed and conditioned it, styling it each morning. It was my security, a big part of how I felt about my appearance. To say I was going to miss it would be an understatement. I had just lost both of my breasts permanently, but it seemed like I was mourning the eventual loss of my hair even more.

It never ceases to amaze me the support and help that come from others when the word gets around that you have cancer. People seem to show up right when you need them. Such was the case when it came to my issue with hair. His name was Mack Fenn, owner of Tantrum Hair Salon. Approaching me one day after Church, Mack mentioned he had experience helping other cancer patients who faced hair loss and offered his help. I eagerly accepted. I knew what a kind, gifted man he was, and I welcomed the opportunity to have his guidance as I approached the unavoidable day when my head would be bald.

I had already decided against wearing scarves. While some people wore them well, I thought a scarf would look ghastly with my small, oddly shaped head. I also didn't want to appear to have cancer, which I soon discovered is a look impossible to escape. But to me, a scarf or hat advertises it even more. I had purchased one of each from the catalog I received at the hospital, but I was definitely leaning towards a wig. I also had to consider my classroom of second-graders. It would be so much easier for them if I could look like the teacher they knew—at least someone with hair.

About two weeks after surgery, before my chemo began, Mack took me to a wig salon. As I walked in I wondered if I would be able to choose from the huge selection they offered. The large room was filled with wigs in every color and style imaginable. The owner took time to explain how wigs were made; the more expensive being hand tied with a lighter, see-through foundation. When held up to the light, you could see through the base. The cheaper wigs were heavier and I'm sure much warmer to wear.

As I walked around the store, I selected several wigs to try on. When I was satisfied I had chosen a sufficient number to begin the process, I sat in a swivel chair positioned in front of huge mirrors. Since I still had my own hair, the lady pulled it all up into a stocking cap. We tried long, medium and short styles and experimented with different colors. I took advantage of this moment when I could see myself as a blond or redhead; spiked, curly, or straight. I began gravitating toward a shorter style closer to my own brown hair and eliminated all but four styles that were the most flattering.

I finally narrowed the selection to a short style that flipped in the back, had light, wispy bangs, and was longer around my ears. The wig was brown, but had a lot of red and blond highlights, bordering on my comfort zone. Mack had me wear the wig outside so I could see it in the sunlight, which made the highlights even more vibrant. It was a lighter brown than my natural hair color, but to order a shade darker would be risky. There were no returns on special orders, so I had to be satisfied with what I could see. Even though it was a sassier style than what I usually wore, and had more highlights than I was conservatively accustomed to, it felt right. I had already taken up a lot of Mack's volunteered time, so I made a decision and closed the deal. I left the store with my new look pinned to a mannequin, and a bag containing wig shampoo, conditioner, and hair spray. The store owner also explained I would need a terry cloth turban to keep my soon to be bald head warm at night. I chose a blue one over breast cancer pink, still not wanting to have any association with the reality in my life.

Driving home, Mack talked about what to do when my hair began to fall out. He spoke frankly, as if it were a normal occurrence, like losing a baby tooth. During my short membership in the cancer club, I observed a trend for women to take control of the situation and simply shave their heads bald when the exodus began. I picked up quickly that Mack had a strong opinion about this. When the inevitable day arrived, I was to call and he would meet me at his salon after hours. Instead of shaving my head, he would cut it very short. There was a chance I may never go completely bald and even a few strands of hair would be helpful in holding my wig in place. It was something to consider as I couldn't picture myself ceremoniously shaving my scalp.

Upon returning home, I was anxious to share what would soon be my new hair style. Kristy was still visiting, and her enthusiasm made me feel confident about my choice. I knew if I got Brittany's approval, it would pass the test as she was my seventeen-year-old fashion expert, and brutally honest. She, as well as my husband, shared their endorsement.

I only hoped they would end up liking the wig on me as much as on the Styrofoam mannequin. It looked kind of cute sitting on my dresser and I felt a sense of power in being prepared. After all, I reasoned, there were some benefits to a wig. Once placed on my head, it took only seconds to gently arrange the locks. No blow dryer or curling iron needed, and get this—it only had to be washed once a month. Wearing a wig would shave off at least thirty minutes of each morning's preparation for the day.

I'm not sure what I was thinking when I decided to go to my hair stylist of ten years and pay money to cut my hair short two weeks shy of it falling out. Maybe I was trying to capture the style of the wig so the transition would be smoother. Perhaps it was my way of feeling in control, like those who chose to shave their heads; or maybe I couldn't stand to see my longer hair fall out when the time arrived. I wasn't usually sure what drove my actions during this perplexing time. My mind was muddled and I often made impulsive and erratic decisions. Whatever the reason, it didn't matter. Long or short, it would soon be gone.

The next hurdle was to prepare my second-graders for the eventual loss of my hair. We were on this journey together and I felt it was better to talk openly than glaze over some of the inevitable and observable effects of cancer. There would be many good teaching opportunities this year and I needed to provide an atmosphere of communication and understanding on a subject that was often feared. The decision to be open proved beneficial for at least one family I know. The mother of one of my students was diagnosed with cancer several years later. She told me about a conversation she had had with her daughter that warmed my heart.

"Were you afraid I might die?" the mom asked her daughter.

"No. Mrs. Bretzing had cancer and she was fine. I knew you would be, too."

I had just returned to teaching after the rocky recovery of my first chemo treatment, knowing it was only a matter of days before my hair would be gone. The children hardly knew me but I couldn't put off the talk I had prepared for them. As we gathered on the rug that morning, I hoped I could phrase my comments in a way their young minds would comprehend. By this time, they all knew I had something called cancer, and there would be many different levels of understanding depending on how much their parents had discussed it with them. I had to assume they knew practically nothing about this disease, so I started at the beginning, attempting to approach the subject through the eyes of a seven-year-old.

"I want everyone to sit up tall and pay attention while we visit together today about something very important. I have missed being here at school with you. Do you know why I have been gone?"

I called on the first hand that was raised. "You have been sick with cancer."

"Right. I want you to know that cancer isn't something I can give you like a cold or the flu. Our bodies are made up of millions of tiny cells and sometimes cells can grow out of control. This doesn't happen very often, but when it does, the bad cells need to be removed, or killed. To kill the bad cells, the doctors give a cancer patient something called chemotherapy which is a medicine. Unfortunately, the chemo, not being very smart, kills the good cells as well as the bad. Some of the good cells chemo medicines might attack are the ones that control hair growth. Since I am receiving chemo to kill any remaining bad cells, it will also kill the cells that make my hair grow. This will cause the hair on my head to fall out. When this happens, at least we know the medicine is really working."

I could tell from their faces most of them were following my carefully thought out presentation, so I continued, "Almost two weeks ago, I received my first dose of chemo medicine, so I will be losing all of my hair in a few days. I want you to be prepared for this. Have any of you seen a person wearing a scarf wrapped tightly around their head with no hair showing? Maybe it was a hat that covered their baldness."

A few hands went up, but no one shared comments, which is pretty unusual for second-graders. I continued, breaking the silence.

"Another option is to wear a wig. Since I will be losing all my hair, what do you think I should do to cover my baldness?" I hadn't planned on pulling them into the decision-making process, but decided at the last minute to give them a chance to feel a part of what I was experiencing.

One of my more outspoken girls shot up her hand. "Yes, Trinity, what do you think?"

"I definitely think you should wear a wig. Then you will look like everyone else."

The room was filled with various forms of agreement, the most I had heard from them since we began our talk.

"Okay. It's settled. When my hair falls out, I will be coming to school with a wig. It will look different than my natural hair, but you're right Trinity, I will look like everyone else. Now I want to hear from you. Does anyone have any questions about what I have told you today?"

After answering their few questions which mostly revolved around the cancer itself, they returned to their desks and the lessons of the day. I felt good about the conversation we had, especially relieved to have the eventual loss of my hair as well as my diagnosis of cancer in the open. I invited them to ask me any questions that they might think of, anytime they wished. After this initial discussion, few ever brought it up verbally, but some would write questions in their daily response journals. These journals, which I titled "You Write to Me, I Write to You", allowed an avenue through which I could respond individually to any concerns. One little girl's grandpa died of cancer and she was especially full of thoughtful questions. I could tell the ones who were thinking about what I had taught them and those who preferred to forget it or pretend it wasn't there. Even at age seven, there are different methods of processing uncomfortable information.

It was a good thing I chose to prepare my class for the eventual loss of my hair because that very evening it began to fall out. I'm not talking strands here and there. I'm talking clumps. The discovery was made when I simply swept my hair aside with my hand. I was amazed how accurate the oncology nurses were in their prediction of the day it would happen, "ten to fourteen days after administration of your first chemo treatment." It was the evening of the thirteenth day. I had to make the decision. Should I try and get through one more day with my own hair or take charge and switch to the wig? I was disturbed with stories I had heard of women washing their hair and coming out of the shower nearly bald. I cautiously ran my hand over my head, only to find a confirming mass of hair entangled between my fingers. Around 8:00 that evening I finally called Mack for advice. He said to meet him down at his salon in half an hour.

After washing my hair and eyeing the situation, Mack said it was time. As he sat me in his chair I looked at the hands on the large clock on the wall. Randy who had come to lend his support, took a picture of the time: 9:00 p.m. I decided I could react to this inevitable event in one of two ways. Either I could become emotional and cry while Mack cut what hair remained on my head, or make light of it and enjoy the moment. With Randy's and Mack's help, I chose the latter.

Mack decided to have a little fun as he cut my hair. He tried different styles along the way to the final destination of one half inch all over. First he cut the sides, leaving a Mohawk which he spiked high. Then he cut everything but the bottom in the back to see how I'd look with a mullet. Randy participated by taking pictures of the entire process. The three of us laughed until tears ran down our faces and I was grateful for a husband and friend who turned a potentially traumatic experience into what it simply was: a very short haircut. I looked like a boy but I wasn't bald.

Mack next showed me how to place the wig on my head properly. Eyeing it carefully, he trimmed it in a few places and magically customized it to enhance my features. After offering some instructions on wig care and tips for future styling, we left the salon.

I was grateful for the selfless time Mack offered in preparing me to enter this phase of life with cancer. I wish I could say I merrily skipped to the car to ride home, but along with my gratitude I felt a big dose of apprehension. My steps were heavy and my mind preoccupied with thoughts of facing everyone at school the next day. It would be obvious that I had reached the moment I had dreaded since I learned I had cancer.

I forced a smile as Randy chatted casually all the way home. I think he was relieved this evening had been lighthearted. Remembering all he quietly dealt with, I tucked my anxiety away and engaged in the conversation, savoring the laughter and relief that another hurdle had been cleared.

Entering our home, I quietly tiptoed past Brittany's bedroom door, hoping to reach my bathroom mirror before she dashed out to see my new look. She never did come out, for which I was thankful. I needed some time alone to study my reflection and analyze my new style. Picking up a hand mirror, I looked at my profile and then the back of my head. It was actually cute from the back. I liked how it flipped across the bottom, giving the hair a playful, impish appearance. The sides covered my ears, some strands having a mind of their own, which added to the untamed look. Staring straight on, I was not as impressed. What was there about this wig that made it look like a wig? With my fingers, I rearranged the wispy bangs to hide the front seam and my short crew cut that threatened to show. Finally deciding to smile at the reflection, I noticed how much better the wig looked. I would have to remember to smile a lot.

Yawning, I carefully removed my hairpiece and placed it on the mannequin. I felt naked and vulnerable, missing the feel of hair on my face and neck. Avoiding the mirror, I searched in my drawer for the blue terry cloth turban and placed it on my head. I lay in bed for a long time, thinking back on the events of the evening, mingled with fear of what tomorrow may bring. If only I didn't have to do this. I finally gave up trying to hold back the tears, silently allowing myself to grieve, but only for a few minutes. There. It was over. I fell into a restless sleep, determined that the loss of hair would no longer get me down.

The next morning, I arose at my usual time to prepare for school. I washed my thinning hair and watched even more of it land on the floor of the shower. Short shavings of hair peppered the bathroom counter and sink. It made a mess and I was glad it wasn't long. I had definitely made the right choice to not wait another day. I finished my routine and after dressing, carefully put my wig in place. Mack had taught me to shake my head after centering it, and then style it with a plastic pick. It was the first day I would emerge into the world wearing my new wig, and I wanted it to look perfect. I spent an unusual amount of time agonizing over the placement of every strand, and was forced to finally be on my way so I wouldn't be late. For someone who was so particular about hair, going into public for the first time wearing a wig was no easy task. I took a deep breath and left the accepting walls of my home to venture out into the often cruel, honest world. I didn't think about it then, but I would have to go through this process again when my hair began to grow back and I weaned myself off the wig. There was undoubtedly something I needed to learn and it had to do with comfort zones, which I was being forced to leave.

As I drove the short distance to school, I kept glancing at my reflection in the mirror on my visor. I didn't like my wig anymore. It looked so different from what I usually saw in the mirror and I wasn't use to my new sassy look. I longed to turn the car around and return home. Sadly, there was no skipping out on school today. My only option was to park my car and walk across that parking lot as confidently as I could. I decided it would be best to at least appear self-assured and go forth with my head held high. As I crossed over to the sidewalk that led to my room, my principal entered the parking lot. Upon seeing me, she slowed down, gave me a thumbs-up and smiled. Sue's approval and support on this monumental day was what I needed right then and I took a deep breath and walked into my room.

When the bell rang for the children to line up and come in to begin their day, a new set of butterflies attacked my stomach. How would they react to my new look? Children are usually brutally honest and I needed to prepare myself for that. I was so thankful for my foresight in taking the time to talk to them the day before, preparing them for this moment. Just in time too. I took a deep breath and opened the door to walk out and greet a chattering class of seven-year-olds.

I don't remember which child asked, but one did have the courage to pop the question. "Is that your wig?" "Yes, it is," I replied with the biggest smile I could muster. This was followed by a general consensus of "Oh-hs" and "Ah-hs" and then back to the normal morning rush of handing me their lunch money, sharpening pencils, hanging up backpacks, and getting drinks before the second bell. That was it. No big deal. I was glad to have the initial unveiling over. I was never more grateful for the mundane morning routine that kept me moving forward like any other day.

As I was helping a few children with their morning warm-up, one little girl came up from behind to ask a question. As she waited her turn, she studied the back of my hair. When I turned to help her, she leaned in close and whispered, "Mrs. Bretzing, you left the price tag on your wig." Startled by what she could possible mean, I felt the back of my head. Finding nothing that resembled a price tag, I thanked her and we continued with the morning lessons. Her discovery was ever present on my mind and I was determined to find the source as soon as I had a break.

After sending the class out for their morning recess, I rushed into the second-grade workroom and asked my two teammates to look at the back of my wig to see if they could find what might look like a price tag. One of them spotted a white tag near the bottom and arranged the wig to cover it. I thanked her; relieved I could at least get through this day without further reference to my price tag. I couldn't wait for the opportunity to snip off the culprit.

My first wig day passed without further incident. The students and co-workers were accepting and kind and we easily went about our daily routine. I realized that there were some things I did have control over, most importantly my attitude. I couldn't choose how my body reacted to chemotherapy but I could choose how I reacted. My choices would greatly impact the children I associated with each day. I owed it to us all to be strong.

Why did I feel compelled to be strong, or at least appear to be strong? Why did I keep so many of my feelings to myself throughout my ordeal, attempting to approach life with a smile and positive attitude? Being optimistic was always easy for me when everything was going well, but I honestly didn't know how I would react when I was diagnosed with cancer. I did know I wanted to do more than just survive. I wanted to survive well and not cower from the trial I had been given.

I didn't want to burden others with my struggles and was determined to maintain my usual optimism, relieving others of the tendency to worry or not know how to react to my circumstances. I noticed early in my journey that my attitude greatly affected those around me, as well as myself. When I found it difficult to be positive, I would pretend to be, resulting in a better day.

The transition from having my own hair to wearing a wig taught me a valuable life lesson. Each day would be miserable if I chose to look inward, focused on my insecurities and how I was feeling. From that very first day when I faced the world without my own hair, I survived by looking outward, trying to help my students and friends become comfortable with my cancer and the resulting side effects.

When I returned home at the end of school and the debut of my new sassy look, I removed the wig in the privacy of my bedroom. Turning it to the inside, I found near the wig's base a white tag that gave the contents, care, and brand name. Not wanting to take the chance of my "price tag" showing again, I cut it as close to the backing as I could and tossed it in the garbage.

From that day on, little reference was made to my wig and the children accepted it without reservation. I attribute this easy transition to the preparation I did the day before, as well as the sweet approval of children. A few times along the way, the children would ask me what I looked like without hair. They were curious, but I didn't have enough confidence in my baldness to remove the wig and give them a peek. I hadn't even shown my own children.

When I reported that my hair was beginning to grow back, my students would sometimes ask how long it was. I would find a boy in the classroom with short hair and reply, "It's about as long as Mark's." The only other time my wig was mentioned was when a new boy moved in and finally got the nerve one day to ask me if I was wearing a wig. I told him I was, and that was the end of the conversation.

Getting use to wearing a wig was not too difficult, but liking what I saw in the mirror was another matter. At times, I felt the color was all wrong. The brightly lit mirror in the staff bathroom at school caused it to look unnatural, accentuating the gold and red highlights. Many times I wished

I had chosen a simple plain brown, only to have someone compliment the rich, vibrant highlights and how they complimented my eyes. My wig's strongest feature was the style and Lauri had her hair cut to match it. The greatest compliment was when my surgeon, Dr. Deyden, exclaimed at my next visit, "Your hair hasn't fallen out yet!" I assured him it had and he was looking at a wig. Even if he was pretending, it was a very kind gesture.

Since the wig was well made, it was light and comfortable. One of its greatest advantages was the little time it took to get ready each day. I would wash my scalp in the shower each morning, apply make-up, eat breakfast, and get dressed. Lastly, I would place the wig on my head, give it a good shake, arrange a few pieces, and be on my way. When I got home, I removed it and placed a hat or turban on my head, just for the sake of comfort. If the doorbell rang, I would dash back to my bedroom and quickly replace my wig. It was usually askew, but better than being caught with no hair which I was extremely sensitive about. I was entering the winter months so I rarely experienced sweating or discomfort and my wig and I finally became a pair.

When I first purchased my wig, I was warned about wearing it when opening a newly run dishwasher or taking something out of the oven. Unlike natural hair, a synthetic wig had the tendency to frizz or even melt when exposed to the slightest amount of heat or steam. To protect my investment, I had developed the habit of removing my wig to cook. I was successful until Thanksgiving.

Two of our children and their families had come for the holidays and were staying in our spare bedrooms. Their presence posed a small problem when it came to wig removal because I wasn't about to let them see me bald. Even wearing just my turban was uncomfortable. Since Thanksgiving dinner was created in my kitchen, I handled the situation by requesting their help in removing items from the oven, and tending to the things cooking on the stove. By avoiding the heat, I could safely wear my wig and still direct the meal preparation. It was the perfect solution, or so I thought.

That evening, upon removing my wig, I discovered it to be covered with a mass of little frizzes. I took some scissors and commenced snipping off the worst of my folly. After about a half hour of trimming the frazzled ends, strand by strand, I finally tired and decided to petition Mack's help in the morning to repair the damage. From that point on, I never wore my wig in the kitchen. It wasn't the last time I almost ruined it, however. As I was ironing one day, I sadly realized the small amount of escaping steam was enough to singe my precious wig again. By this time, I was getting pretty good at cutting off the ruined ends myself.

After my third chemo treatment, I found myself bald except for a grand total of ten or so individual strands that remained loyal. They each stood alone like sentinels that would not submit. Those solitary strands never fell out so I was able to say I didn't go completely bald. They also didn't grow, and being short and stubby with no friends around, they looked pretty hilarious. I thought about their resistance to giving in to the inevitable and considered them an example of hanging in there, despite all odds.

*March 18. 2010*

*Dear Journal,*

*Today I received a call from Sue saying that the artist finished my portrait on our school's Hall of Heroes mural. She suggested I go on campus and see it before school resumed on Monday. It was good advice to get a preview as I can't describe how it felt to walk up and see a life-size replica of me painted on a wall. I have to admit, the artist did a fantastic job. It looked like the old me, copied from a photograph taken in better days. It broke my heart to see Sue's portrait missing. At her request, Sue had the artist remove her image and place me where she once was.*

7

# UNDAUNTED

The next few months of chemo treatments brought difficult times as well as growing opportunities and sweet moments. I was in the middle of a daily struggle to push forward no matter how badly I was feeling. I had finally reached a plateau where I had a better idea what to expect from each treatment and the amount of time needed to get back on my feet. Having settled into a routine fit better into my life style, even if the routine wasn't one I would normally choose. I had resigned myself to the weekly blood draws, doctor appointments, and chemo treatments every three weeks, followed by seven days of shots to repair the damage.

The days in bed after chemo were some of the longest of my life. One way or another I had to figure out how to break the monotony and get my mind on something other than how awful I was feeling. I finally decided to try reading again and discovered that with persistence I could concentrate for small periods on genres that were fictional and uncomplicated.

The trick was choosing the right book. Pulling several selections off my bookshelf, I began a book, tossed it aside, started another, finally settling on a new novel that had just been released titled *The Undaunted* by Gerald Lund. It was a story of the pioneers who settled southern Utah and the trials and hardships they faced. Before beginning Chapter One, I scanned the preface, curious about the author's chosen title. My eyes focused on a paragraph where "Undaunted" was defined.

To be undaunted is "to be unwilling to abandon one's purpose or effort; to be undiminished in courage or valor."

The definition penetrated my heart and I was instantly drawn into the pages of that novel. I reread the meaning of undaunted several times, feeling a surge of energy. I knew immediately that it was exactly what I needed to strive for. It would be my personal motto during my journey with cancer. Even though I lived many years after these brave pioneers, I was also going through a trial that required courage and endurance. My purpose was to rid my body of cancer. I was expending great effort to accomplish this and even though the way was rocky and difficult to travel, I knew I needed to press forward "with courage and valor".

Defeating cancer wasn't my only challenge. It took a lot of self-discipline to continue teaching through the school year. Sometimes after a treatment, it was all I could do to get up in the morning, get dressed, go to school and face twenty-five active second-grade students. I also thought of my progress in overcoming my fear of needles and tests and the unknown still ahead. Yes, this would be my motto to remind me how important it was to face the future with courage and not give up.

I went to the computer and typed out the definition to hang on my refrigerator so I would see and read it daily. I would often run those words over and over in my mind during times of discouragement and they gave me great strength and determination. My friend Lauri took the definition and made me an attractive framed plaque for Christmas that year, one that remains displayed in my home as a constant reminder. I didn't feel it was a coincidence I chose that particular book to read.

Sleep was another problem that escalated as the days wore on. I was becoming more and more sleep deprived which didn't help my general well-being. When I discussed this with Dr. Polowy, he prescribed a sleeping pill which was frequently used with success by many cancer patients. I was told to start with 5 milligrams to determine if that was enough to give me a good night's rest. My daughter Kimberly had taken this medicine before and told me to take it right before I was ready for bed as it worked quickly. She assured me I would sleep soundly and awake refreshed and rested. I followed her advice, but instead of dropping off quickly, I laid there for a good half hour before finally going to sleep. I woke up frequently during the night, not being able to return to sleep easily. If this was to work for me, I clearly needed to increase the dosage.

The next night I took 7.5 milligrams and didn't find it to be much different from the night before. In desperation, the third night I went to 10 milligrams, the highest recommended dose, and slept better than the previous nights. Using this sleep aid, I could catch up on some much-needed rest, but when I went to refill it, my insurance company denied my request. What was I going to do now? I had to sleep or I couldn't function. In desperation, I tried several over-the-counter aids, none of which worked.

At my next blood draw, I explained my problem to one of the oncology nurses. She gave me some samples of a new sleep aid that was available and suggested I give them a try. If they worked, she would call in a prescription. In the meantime, my insurance company allowed my other prescription to be filled and I returned to using the first drug prescribed.

Unfortunately, after a few more weeks of use, this sleeping pill resulted in nights filled with violent nightmares. One of the worst dreams I can remember found me standing before a firing squad. A designated soldier would let go of a heavy wooden beam that would swing straight towards my throat. When the beam stopped, barely touching my neck, the squad would all fire at once, brutally killing me. Then the dream would rewind and repeat, causing me to experience once more the rapidly approaching beam and the horrible sensation of the bullets riddling my body. Becoming more exhausted than ever, I threw the rest of the pills away.

It was time to retrieve the samples the nurse had given me and try something different. Fortunately, they worked and I called the office to see if I could obtain a prescription before the samples ran out. I hit another road block when it was discovered that this new drug was not approved by my insurance company.

I used the samples sparingly, skipping the weekends when I didn't have to rely on a good night's sleep to function at school. As my supply ran low, I resorted to using them every other night and hoped for a solution before I completely ran out. What I didn't know was the nurses hadn't given up. They were familiar with this kind of problem and very good at convincing insurance companies of patients' needs. I found out that one of the nurses had spent a great deal of time arguing with my insurance company, finally obtaining permission to fill the prescription.

Being a new drug, it didn't come in a generic form and was extremely expensive. With the insurance kicking in, it still cost me $75 a month, but well worth it as it conquered one of the most frustrating side effects of the chemo drugs. The following week when I was in the clinic, I thanked the nurse many times for the effort she extended in getting this drug approved for my use. It made a huge difference in my ability to function and feel better when I could get longer periods of uninterrupted sleep.

Not all was lost or wasted during the many nights I was unable to sleep. Being wide awake with the house completely quiet, I found time to reflect on many things. I often thought about the lessons I was learning from this trial. Before cancer struck, I often had my priorities wrong. I was focused primarily on teaching, which required many hours to satisfy my high standards. I absolutely relished teaching and was constantly thinking of new ways to present material and improve my methods. I was concerned about filling the various needs of my students and helping each reach their potential.

There is nothing wrong with being passionate about a job, but I was doing so at the neglect of my personal relationships with my family and even my friends. They often came second and I knew I needed to find a better balance. Nothing was more important than my husband, children, grandchildren, and my mom. Even though I did spend time with family, my thoughts were often on work. I had a hard time letting go of the day as I drove out of the school parking lot. Facing the possibility of a shorter life caused me to carefully consider the path I was walking. I was reminded of what was really important and the necessity of obtaining more balance in life. Too bad it took cancer to jolt me into an evaluation of my priorities.

During these quiet nights when I couldn't sleep, I would often spend time in prayer, asking for understanding, increased faith, and strength to get through the next day. Frequently I would cry out in frustration at the difficult road I was asked to travel. Many times, I uttered prayers of gratitude for the tender mercies being sent my way, usually through others who met my needs and offered encouragement. As a result of turning to my Heavenly Father, I developed a closer relationship with Him. I learned I couldn't go through this experience without His help. I felt of His love for me personally, and received many confirmations of peace. As frustrating as it was to lie awake for hours, I found these moments of communication with God to provide the strength I needed to press forward with faith, despite the twisting road filled with potholes that stretched ahead into unknown distances.

There were times I would listen to my iPod. In the beginning, I chose Christmas music when I thought all my treatments would end the first of December. As I listened, I received encouragement in knowing that when the world was preparing for Christmas, I would be completing my chemo. When my treatment plan changed to well past the holiday season, I abandoned Christmas music and changed to a selection of upbeat music to raise my spirits. One early morning when I couldn't sleep, I had my iPod on shuffle mode and the first song to play was by the Beach Boys with the lyrics, "Don't worry baby, everything will turn out alright." I chose to view it as a little message just for me. Music often played an important role during this time of my life as it lifted my spirits and provided a temporary distraction from my discomforts.

Time slowly passed and it was finally early November. In October, I had shifted my treatments from Wednesdays to Fridays to accommodate the week of parent/teacher Conferences and I had just completed my fourth chemo treatment. Brittany offered to drive me to the hospital on Saturday for my daily Neupogen shot, so we had some time together, which seemed far too infrequent lately. I never felt like doing much after treatments and it took every ounce of energy to fulfill my obligations at school. I felt guilty about this and tried to make the most of whatever time we had together. During the drive to the hospital, we enjoyed visiting and I was grateful we could do something together that day, even if it was only accomplishing the mundane task of getting my shot.

On Sunday morning, Brittany woke up with flu-like symptoms which included a nasty sore throat and muscle aches. As the day progressed, she worsened. Our family physician, Dr. Dinsdale, immediately prescribed Tamiflu and scheduled an appointment for her to be seen the first thing Monday morning. This was the fall of 2009 and there was a nationwide scare about the H1N1 virus, better known as the swine flu. The immunization for that strain of the flu had not been released yet and people were worried. There had been deaths reported, mostly the very young or old, or those with weakened immune systems. On Saturday, Brittany and I had spent considerable time together. Having had chemo the day before, I was at risk of catching whatever she had with my low white blood cell count. I desperately wanted to follow my motherly instincts and care for her, but further exposure was dangerous.

The following scene has played out many times in my mind over the years. Randy, concerned about his daughter and my well-being, scrambled into motion. Being a dentist he had several boxes of latex gloves at home. Putting on a pair and grabbing a container of Clorox wipes, he began sanitizing the house; doorknobs, light fixtures, the entire kitchen. Running back and forth between us he spent the day providing for our needs. After he took care of Brittany, he would wash his hands, put on new gloves and take care of me. Both of us had a bottle of hand sanitizer by our beds which he reminded us to use frequently. I watched in awe as he magnified his role as caregiver, being adamant about keeping us apart. I couldn't help but smile at his meticulousness, and even though he used our entire supply of sanitary wipes, his loving service warmed my heart.

Brittany had a rough night throwing up repeatedly. She was running a fever and coughing. Randy had patients scheduled and had to be at work Monday morning and so my friend Julie took Brittany to her doctor's appointment. After examining her, the doctor wanted Brittany to go straight to the Emergency Room as she was severely dehydrated. Brittany didn't tell us this important piece of information until days later, but instead tried to force more liquids. As we suspected, she tested positive for the swine flu.

Since I was unable to care for her, Julie offered to take Brittany to her home. To fully appreciate this sacrifice one must know that Julie had three children at home, along with a husband, all of whom would be exposed to the dreaded swine flu. Giving no thought for herself and having faith her family would be protected, she grabbed Brittany's pillow and pajamas and was gone before either of us could protest.

Alone at home, I cried. I was greatly touched by the loving service of a dear friend and at the same time devastated that I couldn't help my daughter. Never during this entire journey was I more frustrated at myself for having cancer. I could put up with the havoc it played in my life, but when it came to interfering with the needs of my family, it had crossed the line.

Later that morning, Lauri drove me to get my daily shot. Upon hearing that my daughter had been diagnosed with swine flu, Dr. Polowy prescribed Tamiflu for me. I didn't enter the chemo room, but received my shot in a small room away from the other patients. This flu had everyone scared.

Somehow we made it through the week. On Friday, Dr. Dinsdale received his first shipment of the H1N1 flu vaccine, enough to immunize his staff. He called Randy and I to his office and personally made sure we received the shot, another gesture of friendship and caring that meant so much to our family. Brittany survived a rough week; Julie and her family were spared; and Randy and I escaped as well. What could've been a disastrous outcome was stopped in its tracks by the willingness of others who unselfishly served and provided us with what protection they could.

Shortly after the swine flu episode, I received an e-mail from a reporter of the Mesa Tribune, our local newspaper. This reporter had written an article about a woman who had survived breast cancer and had invited others to share their stories. I responded to her request, wanting to emphasize the importance of not relying on yearly mammograms but doing monthly self-examinations and having any noticeable changes checked by a doctor. It had been several months since I had sent her my story and had forgotten about it. I was surprised to hear from her and even more shocked that she wanted to schedule an interview and publish my experiences for others to read. Her email suggested a time she would like to meet in my home, which happened to be only two days away. In addition, she had arranged for a photographer to come to my second-grade classroom and take pictures while I taught. Not thinking it completely through, I called the phone number she provided and agreed to the interview.

After ending my conversation with the reporter, I began to have second thoughts. Did I really want my story to go public for an entire city to read? I would be allowing others to see me from the inside, which is something I reserved for a few select friends. On the other hand, if someone could learn from my experience and be spared from what I had to go through, it would be worth it. If my story made a difference for even one person, I would be glad I shared it.

I still had misgivings, however, and the day before the interview, I called to cancel. Due to a cold that had worsened I told her there was a strong possibility I wouldn't be at school the day the photographer was scheduled. She wasn't that easy to convince and ended up reassuring me that they could settle for a picture taken in my home. She was determined to do the article and told me she looked forward to seeing me tomorrow. It was apparent I wasn't going to get out of this easily.

Being interviewed by a newspaper reporter was a new experience. I was nervous about saying the wrong thing and having my words twisted forever in print. I wanted to be selective on the amount of information I gave since I knew my students at school and their parents might be reading the article. Due to the location of my cancer, it can be an awkward subject to discuss with all ages and I was feeling quite vulnerable.

When the doorbell rang, it was a relief to see a very pleasant young woman who was kind as well as professional. She was able to put me at ease as I confessed this was my first newspaper interview. We visited for a while as I shared my story and the message I wanted to emphasize about early detection. She personalized the article by asking questions about my family, teaching between chemo treatments, and the feelings I had when I learned I had cancer. I was coughing heavily that day and kept apologizing for the frequent interruptions, but she was patient and understanding. We decided to keep the appointment for the photographer to come to the school and take pictures on Friday, hoping I would make it back by then. It turned out to be a simple, pleasant experience, but I still worried about the contents of the article. It was a sealed deal now so I just had to trust in the reporter's ability to write a piece that accurately represented me and the information I shared.

The article was scheduled to be printed in the Sunday paper. I got little sleep the night before, wondering how this was going to turn out. I was even hopeful that a huge news event might pre-empt my tiny human interest article. At 6:00 a.m. Sunday morning, I could wait in bed no longer. I went outside to our driveway where the paper was always delivered only to find it hadn't arrived yet. It would be just my luck that we had been skipped that morning. I went back to bed, trying to be patient. I checked again at 6:30 a.m., then 7:00 a.m., but there was still no sign of a newspaper. I was tempted to drive around the neighborhood to see if others had received their paper and could almost see myself taking someone else's just to find my article. That would be stooping pretty low, so I decided to eat breakfast and exercise some patience.

It wasn't until after 8:00 a.m. that the paper was finally delivered. Maybe that was the usual delivery time, but I never before had reason to care. Randy went out to get it since it was now daylight and I hadn't bothered to put on my wig. As he brought it in my emotions were all over the place. Mixed with excitement to see the words revealing my story was trepidation in becoming exposed to the public's eye. I hoped I wouldn't be sorry I agreed to this private unveiling.

Tentatively, Randy set the newspaper down on the kitchen counter, removed the rubber band, and unfolded it to the front page. We huddled together and silently began the search, gingerly turning each page with care. I was relieved that it wasn't anywhere in the first section. When we reached the set of pull out ads separating the first two sections, we both saw the article at the same time, positioned unassumingly on the front page of section two.

In bold print, the title of the article read, *Battling breast cancer . . with a smile and a lesson.* Before the article began appeared a subtitle, *Mesa woman stays positive, continues teaching during chemo treatments.* A large photo was included, taken of me reading a book to my students who were sitting on the rug. The shot was natural as I was never more at home in my classroom than sitting in the rocking chair sharing favorite stories with my students.

Reading the article together, I noticed only a few paragraphs mentioning the importance of early detection. The author spent more time on my cancer journey, frequently quoting phrases from our interview. Despite the different twist, it was written well and the information was accurate. It was a human-interest story that others might relate to, but at the same time achieved my goal of encouraging women to act on any changes they may notice in or on their breast. Since the article appeared in October, breast cancer awareness month, the reporter took the opportunity to mention events and fundraisers organized to assist in finding a cure.

Being satisfied that I had made the right decision to share what I had learned from my cancer journey thus far, I carefully snipped out the article. Through the ensuing days, I received frequent comments about the piece, all positive. Not liking the extra attention, I was glad when it was soon forgotten and the school removed the newspaper clipping from the staff bulletin board. The entire experience added some spark to the drudgery often felt with the cancer regimen, but I was relieved when the news became history.

Fall and cooler weather had finally arrived in Arizona. I had completed five of my AC treatments and was feeling the ever-increasing results of the accumulated drugs. My body was wearing down and my energy level was constantly low. It was all I could do to put myself back together after a treatment and teach school. Chemo in its own silent, slinky way was affecting me physically and mentally. Optimism was gradually being replaced by discouragement.

The first day back to school after a date with chemo was always the worst. When I was at my lowest, my second-graders were at their highest level of energy. I had to reset boundaries and expectations. I would no sooner establish a smoothly running classroom according to my standards, and I was gone again for another treatment. Lori, my substitute, faced the same problem when she returned to take over. It reminded me of children with divorced parents, going back and forth between families. My class was getting very proficient in taking advantage of the situation. I couldn't really blame them. They were only children.

What worried me even more was my diminishing enthusiasm for teaching. I didn't look forward to each day as I had in the past. I was beginning to feel like a robot going through the motions and counting the days until the end. I knew I would need to rekindle the spark if I was going to make it through the year. I hadn't even made it through the first semester yet.

It was fortunate that Thanksgiving fell between treatments and I would be able to enjoy my children and grandchildren who were coming for the holiday. As tradition dictated, the event would be at my house, but I would have plenty of help with Thanksgiving dinner. With the promise of family coming for the holidays, I received a needed dose of energy and enthusiasm for life. As the day approached and I purchased everything needed for a proper feast, I found myself in great spirits. I was excited to be with my family and it gave me something to look forward to. Those traveling from out of town arrived by Wednesday evening and thus began a four-day weekend of laughter and reminiscing.

Kristy suggested that after we ate our Thanksgiving feast, we should sit around in a circle and express what we were thankful for. Little did I know this was her plan to announce she was expecting another baby. Her announcement prompted a similar confession from Julie, who was also saving this moment to share her news. Despite the worries and illness cancer brings, we were able to put that aside and rejoice in new life. I was reminded of my many blessings, and the joy the future held.

All too soon, the Thanksgiving holidays passed and the house was quiet again. I couldn't help but think that if I had been able to follow the original plan, my last chemo would be around the corner and I would be done. Instead, I had one more treatment of AC and then five additional treatments of the drug, Taxotere. I was barely half finished with my chemotherapy and it seemed like the road would never end. Despite entering the Christmas season, my favorite time of year, I was depressed with these thoughts.

Each day I was constantly reminded of my baldness. Until I finished my chemo treatments, my head would remain that way. Sometimes between taking off the wig and putting on my terry cloth night turban, I would stare at my reflection in the mirror. It was a sight I reserved for myself, not wishing anyone else to remember me this way. I looked like a little old man with big ears. It made me think of World War II when the Nazis would shave the heads of the Jews in concentration camps. The purpose was to prevent the spread of lice, but I'm sure it assisted in their sickening goal of removing all their victims' dignity and self-respect. Baldness made me feel submissive and vulnerable and I could understand the evil motivation of the Nazis.

To break free of this self-pity, I found the less I dwelled on my lack of hair, the better. I strived to focus my thoughts on the many blessings of owning an attractive wig and other head coverings. I reminded myself that my present condition was temporary. A year from now, I would be back to normal. Most of the time, I was successful in this resolve. I spent fewer and fewer moments alone examining my shiny scalp. I'm glad I remember these feelings, though. Living with the effects of cancer helps me to understand the challenges others face as they tread the same footsteps.

Despite how I felt inside, the mood of the season began to rub off on me. How can one remain despondent when surrounded daily by twenty-five excited second-graders? December days were overflowing with holiday art projects, decorating our room with a tree and lights, and planning the classroom Christmas party. Reading the traditional holiday stories each day added to my growing excitement for this treasured time of year.

With the help of my daughter Julie, I was able to decorate my home like every other year. This was quite an undertaking as I own tons of Christmas decorations and my home goes through a complete transformation. During their visit at Thanksgiving, my son Doug and son-in-law James worked hours to put up our outdoor Christmas lights. This was a great sacrifice of their time, and a precious gift as they knew how important those lights were to me. James spent hours figuring out the quirks in the illuminated candy canes that lined our sidewalk, while Doug hung the icicle lights on the house perfectly even and straight, just like his dad. With that complete, my heart soared with the joy of the season. Even though most of my married children wouldn't be coming this Christmas, Autumn, Ben and their two little boys were still making the trip down from Utah. Adding to the five grandchildren that lived in the area, I would enjoy the magic children brought to this time of year. Realizing how blessed I was, my previous dismal frame of mind was being replaced by contagious Christmas cheer.

Throughout the many years of raising my family, I had developed countless favorite Christmas traditions that meant a great deal to me and my children. I was determined to attempt as many of those traditions as possible. I still had Brittany living at home, and seven grandchildren who would be present for the holidays. I desperately wanted everything to be the same. Despite my lack of energy, I could carry out the most important traditions and find satisfaction in that, but it was necessary to abandon some very dear to me. We didn't make and decorate gingerbread houses. Our Christmas Eve program was less formal and I made far fewer baked goodies. I didn't take the usual plates of cookies and fudge to my friends and neighbors, but I'm sure they understood. I did send Christmas cards, using a year-old family picture, and I never mentioned cancer. Cherished friends living far away never knew of my struggles. I didn't have the heart to use Christmas greetings to convey anything other than tidings of great joy.

The Christmas season was sweetened even more by some mysterious little elves that dropped gifts by our front door each night beginning twelve days before Christmas. I felt like a child again, anticipating each night's clever gift accompanied with a poem. The arrival of each present would be announced by the ringing of our doorbell. By the time we got to the door, the bearer of the gift would disappear into the night so as not to be discovered. I never learned who our elves were. They preferred being anonymous, but the time they took to brighten my Christmas season was truly a gift of love.

I was fortunate in being able to arrange my chemo treatments to miss most of the Christmas season. I had my last AC injection the eleventh of December and was scheduled to get my first treatment of Taxotere on December 29th. I was becoming weary with all the time expended in going back and forth to the Cancer Center. I felt like my car could drive itself there by memory. Chemo, shots, and blood work took time and were constant reminders that my life wasn't normal. I looked forward to having a month, or even a week when I never had to visit a doctor's office or walk into a lab.

I spent the remainder of Christmas vacation recovering from my first treatment of Taxotere. Experiencing an allergic reaction to this drug during my first chemo in August, they were prepared and administered Benadryl prior to the Taxotere. They also slowed the rate it entered my body. These combined precautions worked and I was able to tolerate it. My reaction to this chemo drug was quite different from my experiences with AC. I didn't have nearly the nausea, but I was so exhausted. It was a tiredness that I'd never felt before, a deep down in the bones kind of tired.

New Year's Eve and the first day of the year found me lying around, accomplishing nothing, and I was still dealing with a chest cold and cough. I couldn't help thinking how different this year was than last when my home was filled with family and laughter and I didn't have a care in the world. Now I always felt sick and I had to force myself to get out of bed and press on with my responsibilities. Hope for the future was replaced with depression, anxiety, and a feeling of despair. The next few months were definitely the low point of my cancer experience. I sometimes wonder if my depression was caused from the new chemo drug or from my circumstances. Probably both were equal culprits.

Luckily, Taxotere didn't play as much havoc with my white blood cell count. Dr. Polowy decided to begin with only five Neupogen shots following each dose, instead of the seven I had been receiving. After the fourth shot I began feeling the characteristic bone pain that I had experienced in the past and so I wasn't in the mood to receive a fifth shot. I had to return to school the next day and I knew from experience that if I had too much Neupogen I would either be in pain or have to take pain medicine which would make me too loopy to teach.

Upon arriving at my appointment for blood work and my fifth injection of Neupogen, I explained to the nurse that I didn't want the Neupogen shot. I happened to be dealing with a substitute nurse who was not familiar with me, and she directed my comment to the other nurses. The nurse in charge told her I needed to have the shot. Maybe it was due to my extreme weariness, both physical and emotional, but something in me snapped. I'm usually a very cooperative, easy going patient and would normally have consented to what others thought was in my best interest. I decided that day to be an advocate for my own health and I was going to have something to say about receiving more Neupogen.

With all the calmness I could muster, I explained why I didn't want the shot and appealed the case to my doctor. I told the nurse to ask Dr. Polowy if I could skip the fifth shot due to the discomfort I was already experiencing. I went on to explain that it was just a guess about how many shots I was to receive since this was the first dose of Taxotere. I knew my body and it was telling me that I had reached my limit of Neupogen. I offered to run my blood work upstairs to the lab and when I returned, I would accept the decision of my doctor. I knew him well enough to be confident that he would approve my request if I could just get past the nurses.

When I returned, the nurse informed me that Dr. Polowy said he would let me skip the shot today if my blood work came back with a high enough white blood cell count. If it didn't, I would have to return to the clinic tomorrow for another shot. Agreeing to those terms, I resisted the desire to act smug and left. I felt I had won a small, but significant battle and I was proud of myself for speaking out and not just getting a shot because I was scheduled to receive it. As it turned out, my white blood cells were numerous enough that I didn't have to receive another Neupogen shot. I had been right, and luckily I had a doctor who trusted how I was feeling and listened.

One of the things I remember most about the next four months while receiving Taxotere, was my daily struggle to keep going. The days were long. The nights were longer. It was the longest four months of my life.

I dreaded daytime because I had to get up and be productive. When the alarm sounded, I wanted to pull the covers over my head and stay in bed. Besides being physically exhausted from not being able to sleep, I was mentally frazzled. It was all I could do to make myself get ready for school on the days I went. In fact, it took a great deal of self-discipline, combined with a mental pep talk, to get me into a standing position. Lacking motivation, I showered and dressed slowly, willing myself to return to bed. I remember days when I would sit on a stool and take ten minutes to put on my shoes. Putting my head down into my lap, I would push away the tears, feeling ashamed to be so weak. How was I going to get through a day of teaching second-graders? Each morning was a struggle and I don't know how I got out the door except for the knowledge that there was somewhere I had to be.

I hated nights due to the long hours I lay awake, forced to create solitary thoughts and conversations. Despite the anxiety and work each day brought, I dreaded nights the most. At least in the day there were people and objectives to be concerned about. The nights were lonely as well as long. As I lay there listening to Randy breathe, I was envious of his ability to rest, and even dream.

Then came the week of miracles. Parent Teacher Conferences for second semester had arrived and I had spent hours the previous two weeks putting the final touches on report cards and preparing each student's individual portfolios of work samples. On Sunday, I had reached a low mentally and physically, wondering how I was going to last through this grueling week. In our school district, we are required to teach all day and then conduct conferences after the children have left. We schedule one evening as late as 7:30 p.m., accommodating parents who aren't able to meet earlier. Even in the prime of health, the week is strenuous. Due to my present condition, I knew I couldn't get through the week of conferences alone. I needed a miracle, or maybe several. God provided me with a week's worth, working through other people.

Monday's miracle: I woke up Monday morning feeling emotionally stronger than I had in a long time. I could do this. Before leaving home, I prayed for strength and stamina to face what was required of me. Each parent I met with that day took the time to mention how pleased they were with their child's progress and my valiant efforts to make this year successful, despite my cancer. They verbalized their support and told me they were praying for me. I had five conferences that day, and was reminded five times I was appreciated and a recipient of prayers.

Tuesday's miracle: I had just finished the day's conferences when the mom of one of last year's students entered my room holding a vase of bright pink Gerber daisies. The flowers were beautiful but it was her words that brought tears. "I saw these flowers and they reminded me of you."

Wednesday's miracle: As I dismissed my students for the day, I saw a nicely dressed woman standing outside my room that I didn't recognize. I smiled as she walked toward me, curious as to whom my visitor might be. She introduced herself as Cameron's mom and my mind raced to make some kind of connection. Then I remembered. Cameron was dating my daughter Brittany and had been a big support for her this year. His own brother had been through cancer and he understood what many teenagers could not. Now before me stood his mom, also a teacher at a nearby school. She handed me a frozen yogurt saying, "I know this is a difficult week for you with conferences, and I brought you something to help." I had never met this woman, yet she was thinking of me enough to take the time to lift and encourage.

Thursday's miracle: I wasn't looking forward to Thursday's late night conferences. It was the end of the week and I was physically exhausted. The miracle of Thursday was that I made it through the day and ensuing evening, having the energy to give it my best. It was dark when I ran into my principal near the office after my last conference. Her comments completed my day. "I have seen a few of your parents on campus and each has praised the work you are doing this year. You are a tough lady."

Friday's miracle: I arrived home, elated that I had accomplished the week I had dreaded. Each day's miracle had fortified me to face the next day. As I walked into my home I noticed that my Christmas decorations were gone. My daughter Julie and my friend Lori had neatly packed away all my holiday trimmings. With my limited energy, I hadn't even begun the task of putting away Christmas and at my present rate it may have remained up all year. Deeply touched by the miracles of the week, I sat down and penned this poem, dedicated to the many who daily blessed my life:

*Some say that there are angels*
*Who minister with love*
*That gently guide and help us*
*Back to Him above.*

*But I'm convinced these angels*
*Who serve us without end,*
*Come in the form of people,*
*And you are one, my friend.*

Our loving Heavenly Father is aware of us in our trials and lends support in many ways. I have found it is through individuals who listen to promptings that much of His work is accomplished. One effect of this cancer journey is I've learned how much I want to be that kind of person.

Along with earthly angels, there were times I felt the presence of unseen angels. During some of the lowest moments, most of which occurred at night when I was alone, I would occasionally feel a surge of comfort, love, and support which is not easy to express in words. It always came unexpectedly and would provide me with enough courage to continue forward. One day I was looking at some pictures of ancestors that my cousin had emailed me after our last family reunion. When I saw the picture of my maternal grandfather, an overwhelming impression came and I knew he was one of my comforters. I hadn't even thought of Grandpa Spencer being there for me, as he passed away when I was only six. I had vague memories of his snow-white hair and him sneaking me bites of his pancakes. My mother and I had lived with him and my grandmother during those years before she remarried. The warm feeling of peace and love that I experienced at seeing his picture years later confirmed he was aware of my suffering and was still watching over me. I am convinced the help I received during my darkest moments came from loving family members who had passed on.

I found with cancer, I experienced some of the greatest highs I ever had along with the lowest lows. Despite my week of miracles, chemo was sucking the life out of me, both physically and mentally. If it hadn't been for my teaching job, I probably would have stayed in bed the next four months. I didn't realize it at the time, but I was depressed, a condition I had never before experienced. This new challenge, caused by the different chemo drug, was nearly as debilitating as the flu like symptoms of the previous drugs.

It was during this time that I could have used some outside counseling, but I was too worn out to seek help. I literally had no energy. My previous efforts to be optimistic and undaunted seemed unreachable now. In public I tried to appear as if nothing was amiss and everyone assumed I was doing fine.

I often received words of encouragement along the lines of, "You're looking great!" In reality, I never looked worse. My face was puffy, my eyebrows were only a memory, and it was a waste of time to try and apply mascara to the few eyelashes that remained. My wig was even beginning to look dull and frizzy. That was just my exterior. Inside, I was desperately weary and void of my previous zest for life. I plodded through these months, looking forward to my last session of chemotherapy. The end of March seemed so far away.

Just as I was about to reach my limit of despair, I was granted another bright spot in the gloom of those winter days. It was February, and my friend Peggy called after a long day of teaching. She said there was a meeting in her classroom I needed to attend to help put the finishing touches on the upcoming Family Math Night. I was weary and anxious to get home and wondered why we needed to have a special meeting when it was nearly planned. Reluctantly, I told her I'd attend, hoping the meeting would be short. When I arrived, I was surprised to see Sue, our principal in attendance. That was unusual, but I reasoned she probably wanted to get an update and details of the Math Night.

Since Peggy was the chairman of the Family Math Night, I was surprised when Sue began the meeting. I learned quickly that we hadn't gathered to talk about the upcoming event.

With tears in her eyes, Sue announced the school's decision to add my portrait to the Hall of Heroes mural that welcomed everyone to our school. The school mascot was the Nathan Hale Heroes and the entire wall next to the office displayed a painting of life size everyday heroes. There was a fireman, teacher, astronaut, member of the Armed Forces, Sue, our beloved Principal, Nathan Hale, and now they would be adding me. I was stunned. I definitely didn't consider myself a "hero". I hadn't done anything others wouldn't do under the same circumstances.

I couldn't find the words to express how honored I felt to be a part of our school's Hall of Heroes. As tears rolled down my face, Sue went on to explain my portrait would be completed during spring break in March and the original painter had been scheduled to come from a city in northern Arizona to make the addition. I timidly asked if the artist was going to depict me as I presently looked, but was relieved to hear that she would be using a picture taken before I was diagnosed with cancer as her guide. I left the meeting completely numb with disbelief. This kind and thoughtful gesture came at a time when I needed it most. If the school and community thought I was a hero, I certainly owed it to them to try and resemble one. As difficult as it was to carry on after each chemo treatment, I had to rally whatever strength I could and endure this trial to the end. My second-grade students deserved my best, and despite how I felt, I had a responsibility to deliver it to them.

Another event provided an additional boost during my last few difficult months of chemotherapy. In January, I entered my class in a district writing contest. Each student was to write a persuasive essay convincing The Cat in the Hat to invite their class to his birthday party. Dr. Seuss's birthday, March 3, is widely celebrated by our school district and one of the professional organizations sponsors a birthday party for Dr. Seuss's most acclaimed character, The Cat in the Hat. First and second-grade students all over the district strive to claim a spot at this prestigious event each year. Four different classes are chosen on the basis of their essays and invited to party and dine with The Cat himself. For a seven-year-old, this is a highly coveted experience.

It was a Wednesday in February when I had returned to school following my previous Friday chemo session. I was deep into my math lesson on measurement when in walked a man wearing a tall red and white striped hat, followed by my principal. He carried the book full of persuasive essays we had written and was the bearer of exciting news. Our class had been chosen to attend the birthday party for The Cat in the Hat. Needless to say, that was the end of our math lesson as we celebrated and cheered our success. I had previous classes win this contest, but this year was particularly sweet. Despite the state of my health and the many days I missed, my children had been taught writing well enough to win a district wide contest. It was a moment to cherish and enjoy.

I returned to reality as I learned the date set for this event would be on Friday, March 5. My next scheduled chemo was to be administered on the fifth of March. I didn't want to miss this event with my class, yet I didn't want to postpone my next to last treatment.

After school, I called the number I was given to schedule the bus and explained my dilemma. I was told that the party would be over by 1:00 p.m. and I should be back to school with my class by 1:30 p.m. They would drop us off first so I could still make my appointment at 2:00 p.m., a twenty-minute drive from the school. It would be close, but I was relieved I could still attend the party with my students. I planned for Lori to come and help at the event and then take over after the party, allowing me to leave immediately upon returning to school.

It was a well-organized plan. Unfortunately, as with many well laid plans, it didn't happen that way. As the birthday party was winding down, I could see things were taking longer than anticipated. For example, imagine trying to get one hundred kids away from an exciting event and back on buses to return to school. It's not going to happen efficiently. After cleaning up cake and ice cream, collecting the prizes each child was given, using the bathroom, and counting noses once on the bus, we were running forty-five minutes behind. There was no way I would make my appointment on time and there was nothing I could do about it.

As soon as I arrived at school, I called my doctor's office. I explained I had been on a field trip and we returned to school later than anticipated. Would I still be able to keep my appointment or would I have to reschedule? I had never been late before but sometimes had to wait up to an hour before seeing Dr. Polowy. Despite that, I knew they had strict policies on patients arriving late. I was put on hold to await my verdict.

The nurse returned after conferring with Dr. Polowy and I was told to come. I was relieved I could keep my appointment and not have to interrupt my chemo schedule when I was so near the end. I was also grateful I didn't have to miss the birthday celebration with my class. We had earned this party and it had truly been a day to remember. As small as these tender moments were, each helped to sustain and carry me towards the finish line.

*March 26, 2010*

*Dear Journal,*
*I have looked forward to all of this ending, only to be disappointed that it is not the end.*

*Maybe there is no end.*

8

# THE FINAL CHEMO

Anyone who has had chemo knows how much you look forward to your last treatment. I don't think I looked forward to anything more in my life. I was counting the days. Only one sticker remained to be placed on the chart tracking my treatments. During my many visits to the chemo infusion room, I had been present to witness patients receive their last chemotherapy followed by the opportunity to celebrate. The elated cancer patient got to ring a little brass hand bell followed by all the nurses and patients in attendance clapping. Hugs and congratulations were exchanged. If the patient had enough energy, the ringing of the bell would be accompanied by some dancing with the nurses. Everyone was happy for the lucky individual who was finally done. Soon it would be my day.

The Friday morning of my last scheduled chemo finally arrived. I was planning to teach school that day, leaving a little early to make my scheduled appointment. As I was putting things in order in my classroom before the morning bell rang, the school intercom blared, "Mrs. Bretzing, please come to the office." I couldn't imagine why they needed me. I went grumbling, "This better be quick," as I had a few more things to accomplish before the children arrived.

When I walked into the office, I was shocked to see the entire staff gathered to celebrate my last day of chemotherapy.

I was deeply touched by the outpouring of love and support my dear friends gave, along with a generous basket of gifts, and doughnuts for all. I went around the circle, giving each friend a hug and words of appreciation. It is no wonder I was able to make it through the most difficult year of teaching with the help of the faculty and friends at Hale Elementary.

Upon arriving at the Cancer Center later that afternoon, I went through all the standard procedures of checking in, paying my co-pay, and sitting to wait. Randy went with me and I was anxious to show him the scrap book put together by the hospital's oncology counselor which included photos of artwork and written testimonials from the "Day of Art" held twice a year. I had personally read and browsed through this book several times, bonding with others who had traveled the cancer road. I felt a connection to these people I had never met as I read of their experiences and viewed their feelings expressed through art. This book was an extension of the paintings I had seen on the walls of the cancer floor during my hospital stay when this journey began.

My name was finally called and Randy and I entered one of the familiar exam rooms to wait until Dr. Polowy arrived to check on me before beginning my last chemo treatment. By now I was very familiar with the routine. He would ask me questions, go over my blood work and usually do a physical exam. I always had ample time to ask any questions that came up since my last visit.

Something new had developed since I last saw Dr. Polowy but I didn't think much of it and hadn't even written it down as something to mention. One evening I was sitting on the couch watching a movie when I kept hearing a clicking sound in the wall next to me. It was soft, but distinct and occurred randomly. When I went into the other room, the clicking noise traveled with me, and I realized it wasn't actually in the wall, but resided in my left ear. The best way I could describe it was the sound of gears moving inside a clock as time moves forward. About three days later the random clicking was replaced with constant buzzing, sounding like a field of katydids announcing the approach of dusk. My right ear decided to join the chorus a few days later. Occasionally, the buzzing in one ear would transform into a high pitch ringing for about ten seconds, then return to its previous humming. The clicking would sporadically return, but only in the left ear. I wasn't concerned, but curious about this new phenomenon.

During my appointment, I casually mentioned the buzzing in my ears to Dr. Polowy. I was expecting him to brush it off, assuring me it was just another side effect of chemo. Instead I saw a concerned expression cloud his face and he asked me a few more questions before writing an order for an MRI on my brain. I was completely surprised by his response and countered with, "Surely this is just a result of chemo." He explained that buzzing in the ears was not typically a side effect of the drugs I had been given. In fact, he had never heard of anyone having that reaction from the drugs I was given for breast cancer.

Hearing that I was to have an MRI on my brain to rule out a tumor was like taking a pin and popping all my last day of chemo balloons. I couldn't help but remember my very first appointment with Dr. Polowy and his haunting words: "Breast cancer can spread to the bones, lungs, liver, and brain." It was my final treatment of chemo and I was so excited to finally arrive at this point in my journey, only to receive the disturbing news that I still had another lap to run. So, typical of my reaction to bad news, I brushed it aside and focused on a few questions I had before our appointment ended. I didn't want anything to ruin my long-awaited celebration. During the middle of my chemo, however, I turned to Randy and whispered, "Did you hear what Dr. Polowy said? I can't believe I have to get an MRI on my brain." I could tell that Randy was also shaken by the news.

As I sat receiving the last bags of chemo for breast cancer, I contemplated the many times I had been in that infusion room. No wonder the nurses and front desk receptionists knew me by my first name. I had been there at least once a week for the last eight months which included weekly blood draws, chemo, hydration, and up to seven consecutive days of Neupogen shots. I also saw my oncologist every three weeks right before my scheduled chemo injections and often in between for another prescription for antibiotics to treat an infection. The antiseptic smells were familiar as well as the routine that had been my life for the last eight months. I was grateful it was almost over. I had yet to learn that cancer struggles don't end with the last chemo. It wasn't over, but being naïve to this fact allowed me to celebrate, which every cancer patient deserves.

That day the chemo room emptied earlier than usual. I suddenly realized that I was the last patient in the chair, waiting for my final bag to empty. Out the door, one by one, walked my long anticipated celebration. Even some of the nurses had gone home. As the evening cast shadows through the large windows in the infusion room, I realized my bell-ringing celebration would be as dim as the encroaching dusk.

Remaining were my husband and two nurses to watch me ring the bell. I rang it anyway. It was an empty ring without others around to enjoy my moment, but at least my dear husband, the one that really mattered, was there to relish my victory. "No more chemo", the bell exclaimed. Inwardly, I was jubilant, but outwardly my body was so exhausted from all the events of the day that I was unable to show much emotion.

As Randy and I left the deserted office, I didn't talk. The ensuing brain MRI was a dark cloud hanging over my head. There was too much commotion going on inside to understand my feelings, and so I said nothing. Upon arriving home, I was lifted from my present gloom by a dozen beautiful red roses arranged in a crystal vase. The healthy red petals pointed upward and reminded me of all I had accomplished over the last eight months and the significance of this day. Along with the flowers, Randy presented me with an original poem he composed describing his tender feelings about our journey together. The day I had looked forward to was full of surprises, good and bad. Experience had already taught me that this was the typical pattern of cancer.

*July 7, 2010*

*Dear Journal,*

*Today I bid a final good-bye to my wig. It has been a part of me for the last ten months and despite my disdain for it, I'm grateful for its faithfulness in keeping me from facing the world bald.*

*Walking out of Mack's salon and sporting my own short hair for the first time in months, I experienced a sensation that I never paid attention to before, and wasn't able to sense while wearing a wig. The day was slightly breezy and I could feel the wind on my scalp. Even though it was a warm July wind, I hugged it and danced like a child to my car.*

*I will never take the wind for granted again.*

9

# MY NEVER-ENDING STORY

I remember when I was first diagnosed with breast cancer, I consoled myself by devising a time line. The first date would be my surgery, followed by six treatments of chemotherapy comprising nineteen weeks. According to my calculations, this nightmare would end on December 2 and I could resume my previous life, free of worry, pain, and anxiety. I was so anxious to have my former life back, I never even considered the possibility it may not happen just that way. There was no reason for me to think differently because I had always been in control of my life. I planned and I prepared and in the past, that worked. It ever occurred to me that having cancer meant that things would never be the same again. I heard some refer to it as "the new normal". I refer to it as *The NeverEnding Story*, a favorite movie my children used to watch when they were young.

Reflecting on the pioneer trek of the previous summer, I felt I had reached the top of the mountain only to be so exhausted I couldn't celebrate the victory. Many times during that climb I wondered if it would ever end. Night had obscured any view of my destination so I blindly trudged forward, knowing the upward ascent had to eventually cease. I literally forced my knees to bend, my feet to take another step. Giving far more than I ever thought I had to give, I reached my goal and collapsed. I was hungry, but food didn't satisfy, so tired but I couldn't sleep. My journey was not over and I had to face another day, physically drained. I reminded myself that I did survive the three-day trip, and I learned I was stronger than I realized. The analogy between this experience and my current journey with cancer gave me hope in my ability to conquer seemingly impossible tasks.

Having reached the summit of my prescribed chemo treatments, my mind was just beginning to process all that I had been through. Remember how I stuffed everything I couldn't handle into a file to deal with later? Later had arrived. The cancer folder that I had successfully stashed away, spilled open abruptly, uninvited. I found myself forced to come face to face with my losses: my breasts, my hair, my eyelashes, and my zest for life. I wanted to feel joyful now that my body was free of chemo and breast cancer, but to get there I had to go through all the steps of mourning. Few people understand this. I didn't and I was not prepared.

After about a month of trying to figure myself out, I decided I needed some help. I was thumbing through my chemo handbook when I came across a page of names to call for support. I recognized the name of the hospital's oncology counselor and even though I had never met her, many had spoken highly of her services. She was also recommended by my oncologist when I began having some depression towards the end of my chemo treatments. Typical of my usual hesitation to admit I needed help, I never called her.

This was different however, and bigger than I could manage. I vowed to contact her and set up a time to visit— tomorrow. I couldn't call her on a day that I was depressed because I wouldn't be able to talk to her without crying. So, I would always wait for the next day to call, only to find I was feeling much better. When I was feeling myself, I found it hard to call since I finally had things under control. Why bother when there were certainly many others that needed her more? When I finally placed a call to Patricia, I found her to be a compassionate listener and took her up on her invitation to come to the next breast cancer support group meeting. It turned out to be one of the best steps I took to assist in my healing and I wished I had not waited so long to make that call.

When my chemotherapy sessions ended, I naturally expected that my physical self would regain normalcy. The effects of injecting strong drugs into the body for eight months cannot be reversed overnight. I could see it would be a gradual process and I would have to dig deep to come up with still more patience. I began to look better since I wasn't being injected with the poison that killed my cells and made me feel lousy, but my inner self still struggled with fatigue, aches and pains, and buzzing in the ears. My doctor surprised me when he said the side effects from chemotherapy could last up to a year. That turned out to be a modest estimation. Some discomforts disappeared while others remained.

In addition, when the chemo was over I inherited side effects that I never experienced before. I was feeling numbness and tingling in my feet, which intensified by the amount of time I needed to stand, teaching school. For the entire school year, I hadn't taught more than two weeks at a time. During the last two months of school when my treatments were completed, I was going straight, with no breaks. After about three continuous weeks on the job, I was pooped. My legs and feet were affected most and the tingling and numbness added to the discomfort. On top of that, sleep was still a problem and I had to continue using sleeping pills in order to get a decent night's rest.

With breast cancer, treatment doesn't end when the chemotherapy sessions are over. Many patients must endure a regime of radiation and all hormonally responsive breast cancer patients are prescribed a drug for five years. As I neared my last chemo appointment, I asked Dr. Polowy if I would need radiation. I was elated to hear that radiation wasn't in the plans, but surprised since many of my new friends had to endure these treatments. I considered it a blessing I didn't have to go through daily radiation appointments, along with the unpleasant effects they can cause.

Another side effect that was unique for me was the loud buzzing in my ears. As I mentioned earlier, on the day of my final chemo, Dr. Polowy ordered an MRI of my brain to make sure the buzzing wasn't caused by a tumor. Luckily, the test came back negative. To further pursue a cause, he sent me to an ear, nose and throat specialist who checked my hearing, examined me, and told me there was nothing he could do. It might go away, it might not. It was most likely caused by chemo treatments and the only cure that might work was medication that came with a long list of side effects. I turned that down as I wasn't anxious to be on more medicine, especially one with side effects to cure the side effects. It looked as if I would have to deal with the buzzing, and so like everything else that I couldn't do anything about, I grew to accept it as part of my new life, hoping that someday a cure would be discovered.

As the weeks passed, I received no relief from the constant sound in my ears. Some days the noise was softer than others and I was more successful at ignoring it. Most days, however, the buzzing blared and I had to work at tolerating this annoying souvenir from chemo. Many nights I would wake up in the quiet of my home and the buzzing would be louder than ever. I often wondered if it was the relentless racket in my ears that woke me.

One day when I was going through some of my cancer paperwork, trying to decide what to throw away, I came across a card introducing our hospital's Cancer Care Coordinator. How did I miss that? It's interesting that what was once just another piece of paper becomes a treasure when you need it. I read the pamphlet which said, "Our Cancer Center is pleased to offer our patients the complimentary services of a dedicated Cancer Care Coordinator to help make each patient's cancer journey as stress-free as possible." Under the six reasons why I needed a Cancer Care Coordinator, it stated "Guide you through the wide array of treatment options and support services offered at the Cancer Center." I wondered if this coordinator could help me with this unique side effect I was experiencing. Maybe she had heard of others with this problem which might lead to a solution. I decided to give her a try and sent an e-mail that very day. I explained my dilemma and what had been done already to try and find the source of the problem and perhaps a cure. I also wrote that I had read in a recent Health Magazine that some people with tinnitus (phantom noises in the ears) had found relief through massaging and manipulating bones in the head. This often takes pressure off the ear's auditory nerves. Perhaps one of the hospital massage therapists was familiar with this approach and could help me. After making my plea for any small thread of advice or help, I logged off, hoping to hear back in a few days.

The next afternoon I checked my e-mails, wondering if Candace, the Cancer Care Coordinator, had answered me. How surprised I was to find that she had not only answered, but had done it within five minutes of my original message. She was very helpful and understanding and asked me to send her the names of my chemo drugs so she could research the companies for this possible side effect. She also said she would have the head massage therapist in the hospital call me. I couldn't believe I was getting such a quick response to my request. Sometimes all we have to do is ask.

The very next day Theresa, the massage therapist, called and invited me to come in that morning. I was already out on errands, but decided to swing by the hospital and try my first massage. It wasn't on my list of plans for the day, but I hated to turn down an opportunity, especially when both she and Candace were so motivated to try and help. When I arrived, she was free to begin and so I sat down after introductions. We decided it was best to remove my wig so she could massage my head properly.

Theresa had an amazing touch. With her hands, she gently rubbed my shoulders and neck and then traveled to my head. As she massaged my temples she asked if it felt alright, not wanting to irritate me in any way. I told her it felt wonderful. I relaxed even more as she continued to rub the bones in my head, on top, behind my ears, and the back of my neck. I marveled at her ability to put me at ease and gently, ever so gently, work at solving my problem.

When she was done, I still had the buzzing just as before, but neither of us expected it to go away immediately. She invited me back for another session and said she would teach me how to do it myself. She would also do some research and look for additional techniques she could add that might work. I was filled with gratitude at her willingness to help with something that left the doctors baffled, and me, frustrated. Even if it didn't work, at least an attempt was being made and that in itself was comforting.

A week after my first meeting with Theresa I was back in her office for another session. I was looking forward to her magic touch that might eventually lead to relieving the demon in my ears. Perhaps she had contacted some of her colleagues that had clients with this problem and they would shed some additional light.

When I arrived, I sat and concentrated on relaxing as she lightly touched my head and used the heat from her hands to heal. As she finished, I asked if she had the chance to talk to any of her friends who might help. She had, and I was crushed as she told me that nothing worked, except time. If the patient was one of the lucky ones, he or she would wake up one morning with the problem resolved. Again, I hit a brick wall and all my hope for an escape came down to being patient and waiting for it to hopefully go away. As I write this, the buzzing is still present, but my ability to cope has increased. What else can I do? After six years of constant buzzing, it has become the norm.

You may be asking yourself by now, what about my hair? Was I noticing some growth? I surely must be looking forward to the very best part of reaching the end of chemotherapy. I am happy to report some exciting developments in this department.

When I was finished with my first set of chemo drugs and beginning the Taxotere, my hair slowly began growing back, only one couldn't really call it hair. I would describe it more like peach fuzz. It reminded me of my own sweet babies as they began to grow their heads of hair. Peach fuzz or hair, something was finally happening. I quickly changed from the cheap shampoo I was using (yes, I did shampoo my scalp) to an expensive name brand. My new beginnings needed the best there was to offer.

As I received my five final chemo treatments, I began to see gradual progress on my head. When it was close to one half inch long, I noticed that the straight hair that I was accustomed to was replaced by tight curls. It was so curly that I would have to stretch the strands to see the correct length. I had heard that this could happen and since I loved natural curls, I was ecstatic. It was coming in thick too, and it wasn't long before my whole head was covered with soft curly locks.

It was all so perfect, except for one thing. The color. Whereas I had some gray hair which I colored professionally before chemo, I was now entirely gray. I wasn't ready to emerge from this experience looking years older, and I had read that it wasn't good to color hair for six months to a year after having chemo. I had also read that it wasn't uncommon for hair to come in a completely different color, like red or black. Why would mine have to be gray? Gray made me look so washed out and ancient.

When I met with Dr. Polowy for my evaluation appointment after my final chemo treatment, one of my first questions was, "Can I color my hair?" If he told me, "No, you need to wait awhile," I'm not sure if I would have listened and followed his counsel. I was so against being gray. I remember an acquaintance of mine who had beautiful black hair. After enduring chemo for breast cancer, her hair grew in completely gray. She decided to go with the gray, and looked great, but it wasn't for me. I can't tell you how relieved I was when Dr. Polowy said it would be fine to color my hair. What a great guy. I wanted to hug him at that moment. I was so relieved I had the go ahead to wash away the gray.

I decided to let it get a little longer and stronger before I took the plunge to color my new locks. I set a target date for this big event. It would be July 7th, the one-year anniversary from learning I had cancer. By then, my hair should be almost two inches long and I could finally get rid of my wig. Since the hot Arizona summer months were approaching, I was not going to miss wearing it.

Waiting for hair to grow is like watching a pot of water get ready to boil. Every night I'd stand in front of the mirror and straighten the curls to note any progress. This nightly routine probably stunted the growth. By watching it so closely, it never seemed to change. I was certain it had stopped altogether. I also noticed that some areas grew faster than others. The hair on top of my head and along the neckline was almost two inches long by my target date in July, but the hair along my forehead was barely one half inch. Since I've worn long bangs my entire life, I would have to become accustomed to this new look.

I had days where I could hardly wait to ditch the wig and I wanted to move the hair appointment with Mack closer. Then there were other days that I thought it might be better to have it grow longer before coloring it. I didn't want to do it too soon, especially since my hair still had the texture of a baby's fine locks. Even with all the inner debating I stuck to my original appointment date and continued to wait as patiently as possible, while measuring the growth each night.

About two weeks before my hair appointment, I started wearing my wig less and less. The weather in Arizona had changed from hot to extremely hot, and now that I had a layer of hair on my head, the wig was almost unbearable. I would wear the wig whenever I left the house, but as soon as I got home, off it would go. On top of it being suffocating to wear, it was also looking rather scraggly and unkempt, and was missing its original sheen. Time had taken its toll on my hairpiece. My appointment couldn't come soon enough.

The night before July 7, I took my wig off for the final time and placed it on the Styrofoam mannequin. There was no looking back. I was anxious to be myself again and take the next step in my recovery. The following morning, I washed my hair but instead of donning my wig like I had done every morning for the last ten months, I arranged my curls with my fingers and prepared for my appointment. I decided to go without my wig, even though my hair was gray. It was an early morning appointment so the chances of running into anyone I knew were slim. I was wrong about that. As I parked my car and began walking down the sidewalk to the entrance, an old friend came out, witnessing the gray hair that I had carefully hidden from the world. Diplomatically, she didn't remark on the color, but was amazed at all the curls and excited that my hair was growing out. She wished me luck and I gingerly entered the salon.

Mack was ready for me and he began by washing my hair again with a shampoo that is used before applying color. There was some discussion on what color to prepare since I wanted to go back to my original medium brown, which was darker than the wig I had been wearing. Mack didn't want it to be too much of a difference and so we compromised. I'm glad I listened to him because it took me some time to adjust to the darker color. I had been seeing myself either light brown with highlights, or gray for months.

After applying the color, Mack trimmed a few places that had grown uneven and showed me some styling tips. Styling amounted to applying a small amount of gel and arranging the hair with my fingers. He advised against using a blow dryer as that would cause frizzing. Right now, it was best to go with the natural curls and enjoy them. I intended to do just that.

Driving the short distance home, I was anxious to be in my own bathroom and get a good look at my real hair. The style and color were different than I had been wearing for the last ten months and I needed some time to adjust. As I stared at the reflection in the mirror my heart sank. The color seemed too dark. I had asked for it to be darker than my wig, but the change seemed dramatic. My hair was too short to highlight, so it was all one color. While the wig had had too many highlights for my taste, now I had none.

It took only a few days to adapt to the color, but it took much longer to be comfortable with having no bangs. I could pull a little hair down on my forehead, but it was so short it looked ridiculous. Not having hair on my forehead reminded me of little children who cut off their bangs and have to deal with it until the hair finally grows out. Being curly made them seem even shorter.

Trying to remain positive, I examined the other areas of my head. From the crown of my head down through the back and sides were a mass of curls which I enjoyed immensely. It was easy to style and I knew I was going to enjoy the curls as long as they remained. I had been warned that as time passes hair returns to its original state, which in my case would be straight. Sometimes the curls would last a few months, or if luck would have it, a year. I was definitely going to enjoy this one and only bonus from chemo as long as I could.

The real test was going out in public with my new look. I was self-conscious and I had to adapt, just as I did with the wig. The whole process was made easier by leaving town. Seriously, no sooner had I shed my wig then we were packing our bags for a vacation. We were visiting family in Utah and thankfully my family tends to be very gentle and supportive. They didn't see me on a daily basis and so the change wasn't as abrupt. They loved my new look and with their support and the passing of time, I also accepted what I saw in the mirror. With practice, I learned to work with all the curls and by the time I returned to Arizona, it had grown another whopping half inch.

I finally began to look at myself as appearing normal again and wasn't self-conscious as the new school year began. At our first staff meeting, Sue asked each of us to stand and share something we had done during the summer. When it was my turn, I commented, "I spent the summer growing my hair." Sue replied, "Doesn't she look great!" Her comment was followed by clapping and many congratulations. I had cleared another hurdle in my cancer recovery, and with each achieved hurdle came more confidence in my ability to cope emotionally.

As the year progressed, my hair continued to steadily grow. I received many comments on how curly, thick, and healthy it looked. My hair stylist was surprised how evenly it was growing and had to trim it very little. I was always reluctant to cut off even the smallest amount when I went in for my appointments. I savored every inch of growth as if the effort to get it to its present length was some great accomplishment.

By Christmas of that year, my hair was finally at a length that appeared normal. It was short, but many people wore it that way, and I was still enjoying the natural curls. A day didn't go by that I wasn't grateful for the healthy, thick hair that covered my once bald head. From my association with other cancer patients, I knew not everyone was that fortunate.

As the one-year anniversary of my wig removal approached, I was overcome with gratitude as I gazed in the mirror at my full head of hair. The curls still remained, which I loved, and the color was perfect. The next year, my second anniversary, I still had a thick head of curly hair, which had been trimmed many times. As each month went by and the curls lingered, I felt so grateful. My hair continued to be easy to maintain and style. Six years later, I can report that the curls are still present. They have loosened, but I can still get away with scrunching my newly washed hair and letting it air dry. It's been fun for someone who previously had straight hair.

Before being diagnosed with cancer, I never experienced an overdose of anxiety, but chemo treatments changed that. For whatever reason, I found myself facing many sleepless nights suffering from anxiety attacks. If I woke up in the night, I could expect to drift into fretful thoughts and worries, unable to return to sleep for hours. I worried about the silliest things: *Was it time to change the oil in the car? Did I lock the front door? When I answered Mary's question, did I say the right thing?* These trivial concerns would keep me awake far into the night. I tried several brands of sleeping pills but found that taking a small dose of anxiety medicine before bed helped the best. I didn't wake up groggy, and it relaxed me enough to get at least six hours of worry free sleep. Sometimes I would wake up when the medicine wore off and was tempted to take another dose so I could get some needed rest, but I resisted, trying to avoid more dependence on it.

For at least a year after my last chemo, I had anxious moments whenever anyone asked me to do something out of my daily routine. I felt I could only handle so much and would often turn down anything that required more than teaching school and maintaining my home. I wasn't use to saying "no" to people, but I learned the importance of doing so. As I look back, I wish I hadn't felt so guilty about this. I was certainly entitled to take some time to regain my strength. I appeared to be well and healthy which was what I wanted, but most people had no idea how I felt or how very much I had been through since I only shared it with a few. I simply hoped they would understand and be patient. As time passed my energy and abilities gradually returned and as they did, I took on more responsibility and opportunities to serve.

People often laugh at the mention of "chemo brain", a condition that is actually real. I don't know the mechanism of chemo brain. I wonder if the doctors even understand it. Maybe it is the effect of drugs playing scramble games with the brain cells. During the months when drugs were being pumped into my system I found that I couldn't express myself clearly. I would completely forget everyday words or even worse, I would pause in the middle of a sentence, failing to remember what I was talking about. This malady showed up often in my teaching, but second-graders are not critical, even if they did notice. It was most frustrating when I would forget how to spell a simple word, so I compensated by not writing words on the board. One day I was helping a student write a poem and she was trying to find a word that rhymed with "fire". She had chosen "liar", spelling it "lire". It didn't look right, but for the life of me I couldn't think of how to spell it correctly, finally sending her back to her seat with the incorrect spelling. The spelling of "liar" finally came to me that evening, out of the blue when I wasn't even thinking about it.

Months after my final chemo treatment, I still struggled with these problems, but not with the same intensity. The incidents came less frequently, but I still had difficulty when it came to reading and following directions. Comprehending nonfiction was especially difficult as I couldn't remember details or specifics. Not wanting to be obvious about this deficiency, I tried to avoid continuing education classes offered by our district, and especially the need to follow written directions.

The first year after completing treatment, I was placed in charge of the Stanford Testing materials for my second-grade team. This involved attending a meeting where procedures were explained and detailed directions given which included: how to count and separate the tests for each class, how to administer the tests, and what was expected when the tests were collected, counted, and bundled for return to the school district. I came away from the meeting with a folder filled with colored pages of detailed directions such as "before testing", "during testing", and "after testing". My head was swimming with all the information that had been imparted and I tossed the folder on my desk, hoping that I could process things better on another day.

With considerable effort, I managed to explain the "before testing" information to my team at the staff meeting the following week. I was relieved to get through the first set of directions enough to teach the others what to do. "During testing" had minimal directions and since I was familiar with testing procedures, that section didn't cause any concern. It was the "after testing" directions that got the best of me.

This section consisted of multiple pages of step by step procedures for the correct handling of testing materials that had to be followed perfectly. I would read each direction several times before attempting the required task. I was in a room with other teachers doing the same thing for their grade level, and I noticed they were taking only a few minutes to finish the job and leave. I was struggling with every step and ended up in tears over this simple assignment. I finally gave in and elicited the help of another teacher on my team to assist me in finishing the "after testing" procedures. There was no way I could accomplish this in a timely manner without support. I was worried that my principal might think I wasn't capable of teaching if I couldn't complete such a simple assignment. I explained to her that my creative side hadn't been affected by chemo, but when it came to technical issues, I was a bundle of anxiety. She understood and the next year, gave another teacher on my team the responsibility for handling the testing materials.

The good news is that as the years have passed, my ability to process directions and remember facts has increased. What a relief to find that chemo brain isn't a permanent condition. Anxiety has markedly decreased as well, and my ability to concentrate and remember has improved. I thought the duration of chemotherapy was long. Confronting and conquering the emotional enemies I faced has taken considerably longer.

*August 17, 2010*

*Dear Journal,*

*I just walked in the door from my appointment with Dr. Shaw, the Endocrinologist. He seems very knowledgeable, and having been referred by Dr. Polowy, I trust his judgment. I consented to a biopsy of my right thyroid but fear what he might find. Knowing that a PET scan and ultrasound both showed evidence of a problem has me worried.*

*I'm not ready to face cancer again.*

10

# NEW CHALLENGES

August 2010 signaled the beginning of a new school year and a fresh start. The students were last year's first graders and most of them were unaware of my struggle with cancer. They didn't see me as Mrs. Bretzing with cancer, but simply as their teacher who came every day to help them love to learn. Many of their parents were also oblivious of my past, or at least politely never mentioned it. They accepted my short hair as a style preference, not as my best alternative to recent baldness. It was genuinely refreshing to have a new beginning.

I was also teaching with two new second-grade teachers who only heard whisperings of my past. We could develop a normal relationship based on now, not what was. I was determined to make it a good, healthy year and return to being my old, happy, motivated self. My body didn't match my mind, however, and the first semester of school brought two new surgeries accompanied by more doctor appointments and pain. I apparently needed more practice refining the traits of patience and endurance.

With the end of chemotherapy the previous March, I began having trouble with my feet. Both heels hurt whenever I walked which meant they hurt most of the time. I stopped wearing shoes with backs and resorted to sandals which were perfect for the upcoming summer months. My right foot was the most painful and I eventually visited with my primary care physician for advice. He examined the troubled areas and concluded that I had heel spurs, prescribing an anti-inflammatory to help with the pain.

Right after his diagnosis, I left for Utah to spend some time with my children and help with Kristy's new baby, due in July. I soon discovered the medicine did nothing for my pain, which was worse when going up and down stairs, a daily necessity at Kristy's house. As time passed, I couldn't walk without limping and my right heel became swollen. I decided I needed to get the opinion of a specialist when I returned home, and luckily I knew a good podiatrist. The problem was fitting a doctor visit into my tight schedule. I had a lot to accomplish with summer ending and the new school year beginning.

Dr. Allen looked concerned as he examined my feet. He took X-rays of the affected areas and left me alone to ponder the problem while he examined the pictures. Upon returning, Dr. Allen gently stated, "Unfortunately, there is no conservative answer to what has happened." He showed me the X-Rays and the calcified mass that had separated from my Achilles tendon. Although it was evident in both feet, it was more pronounced and advanced in the right foot. The only option was surgery and removal of the mass, cutting the Achilles tendon and then repairing it. He suggested doing the right foot first and the left foot after the right completely healed. Was this a side effect of chemo? Dr. Allen didn't think so, but it sure chose an interesting time to manifest itself.

At first I was opposed to another surgery. It was someone else's turn to support the medical field in their profession. I was more than ready to resume my previous status of "excellent health". I worried that others might think I hadn't completely conquered cancer if they found I was going in for more surgery. A day didn't go by when I wasn't asked how I was doing or feeling, which I accepted as sweet gestures of concern and kindness, but I wanted to wash my hands of the stigma of being "sick". It would be hard to hide foot surgery. I would need to wear a heavy black boot for a minimum of four weeks. I was still looking forward to a full month when I didn't have to go in for a doctor's check-up, port flush, or blood draw. Surgery was the last thing I wanted.

Unfortunately, my feet weren't the only health problem I was facing. The time had arrived to investigate the spot found on my thyroid during my initial PET scan. Dr. Polowy had sent a referral to an endocrinologist. Heavy on my mind was the possibility of tackling another cancer.

The appointment with the Endocrinologist was in August, just a few weeks after meeting with the Podiatrist. I felt I was juggling two different health issues when all I wanted was to return to my previous healthy existence. I decided not to worry about possible thyroid cancer because Dr. Dinsdale felt it was probably a benign nodule found in many women's thyroids.

Upon examination, the Endocrinologist, who I will call Dr. Shaw (not his real name), also felt that it was probably benign but wanted to biopsy it to be sure. Of course he only performed biopsies in the mornings, requiring me to miss a half day of school. Missing school was exactly what I was trying to avoid this year.

Having endured biopsies on both my breasts, I was calm when I arrived at my appointment. As I positioned myself on the exam table, I was surprised when Dr. Shaw entered and prepared to begin. Expecting to receive local anesthesia before samples were obtained, I was rather surprised to learn that numbing was not the standard procedure before performing a biopsy on the thyroid. Dr. Shaw assured me it would be quick and patients tolerated it quite well. I trusted his opinion and tried to be brave as I saw six-inch-long needles pass by my range of sight. As he inserted each needle, I felt the probing instruments search for the needed tissue samples. It wasn't comfortable, but I endured it, remembering his promise that it wouldn't last long. Dr. Shaw used an ultrasound to guide him and was finally satisfied with four pokes. When he announced he had what he needed, I let out a sigh of relief, thankful the procedure was over. I would hear the results in a just a few days, and since I wasn't worried, I put the events of the biopsy in the back of my mind.

In the meantime, I decided to go ahead with foot surgery during my October break from school. I would have a full week to recover and the only day I would miss would be the Friday before when surgery was scheduled. Having two full weekends to heal was a plus and I was confident that all would progress smoothly and I could return to school without a glitch. Most people wouldn't connect my surgery to cancer, which couldn't be proven anyway. It was probably just a coincidence that it occurred after eight months of chemo.

I scheduled surgery on my right foot for Friday, the 8th of October. Lori agreed to substitute on that day and I made all the necessary arrangements, including putting my grades on a flash drive so I could fill out report cards at home during Fall break. When we returned, it would be parent/teacher conferences and report cards needed to be completed by then.

It had been a full week since the biopsy on my thyroid and I hadn't heard from the office concerning the results. From past experience, I determined that was a good sign. I decided to call anyway and left a message for them to call me with the results of my biopsy. I received a call back that very day assuring me that I didn't have thyroid cancer, but Dr. Shaw wanted to see me the following Monday. I couldn't imagine why he felt a follow-up visit was necessary, except perhaps to explain the results. He had so few openings that I was surprised they could fit me in. It was odd and something I wondered about throughout the weekend.

As I innocently met with Dr. Shaw the next Monday, I listened intently trying to figure out exactly what he was saying. Was I hearing him correctly? His nurse had told me over the phone last week that I didn't have cancer, but he was telling me that there was a possibility I did. The biopsy wasn't conclusive and the only way to rule out cancer was to remove the right thyroid. If I chose not to have surgery, I would be required to come in for an ultrasound every three months to keep an eye on the tumor.

I sat speechless, trying to digest this unexpected news. Whatever made me think months earlier that as soon as chemotherapy was complete, my life would magically return to normal? Clearly, I had no idea the potential impact cancer can have on the lives of its victims. The celebrated last day of chemo is certainly one milestone to achieve, but depending on the individual, the cancer effect can extend far beyond what was ever expected. I wasn't prepared for this, yet maybe there is no way one can prepare. I felt like my efforts to be optimistic were constantly under attack and it took all the strength I could muster to not let a new threat of cancer drag me down.

Feeling once again that my body had betrayed me, I stared at my doctor as he went on to recommend a thyroid surgeon. He asked if I had any questions, and consistent with my inability to think clearly in the moment, I shook my head. Stunned at what had transpired in the last fifteen minutes, I walked out of Dr. Shaw's office, hardly noticing the stifling August heat. Driving home, I decided to remain quiet about this surgery, allowing my friends to continue to rejoice and believe my struggles were over.

I made an appointment to meet with the recommended thyroid surgeon for the first week after my foot surgery. It would still be fall break from school and Randy had the day off so he could go with me. Meanwhile I had to concentrate on preparing for end of quarter report cards, lessons for my substitute, and surgery. I attempted to get everything in place around the house, even though I had been assured I would be able to put weight on my foot with a walking boot after four days. I was expecting the recovery to be easy and quick.

With so much to accomplish, the day scheduled for my foot surgery arrived quickly. I had just completed my first quarter with a wonderful class of second-graders, and was looking forward to a good year. I didn't mention my upcoming surgery to my students, or to many of my friends. I wanted this to take place quietly, absent of fanfare or attention. I was looking forward to having less pain in my right foot and having the ability to walk without limping. It would also be nice to wear many of the shoes sitting idle in my closet. I wasn't prepared for what really took place.

When I woke up after surgery in the recovery room, I was in so much pain that tears filled my eyes. It was the worst pain I had ever felt. I never knew how uncomfortable foot surgery could be, especially when a bone or tendon is involved. After leaving the hospital, my husband drove me straight to my mom's home to borrow her wheelchair. There was no way I could put any pressure on that foot, even in a walking boot, and I wasn't given crutches. My first night at home was sleepless as the pain medicine I was prescribed didn't come close to relieving the intense pain. This was a bad start to my expected speedy recovery.

I spent the entire week of my fall break from school in a reclined position, recovering from surgery. As I neared the end of the week and the pain hadn't lessened, I wondered how I would be able to stand all day when school resumed on Monday. It seemed improbable, if not impossible. Even with the walking boot, I was unable to put weight on my right foot. We finally solved the dilemma by renting a scooter made for foot and knee surgeries. It helped immensely to be able to rest my leg from the knee down on a padded cushion and use my good left leg to push me where I needed to go. It worked well, but was a bit tricky maneuvering around the desks at school. I used it for one week, but wished I had rented it for three weeks. I would soon find out this surgery was going to take far longer than average to heal.

My Podiatrist was apologetic and surprised at my slow recovery. Perhaps it was the condition of my weakened body that kept the bone from healing within a normal length of time. The surgery didn't accomplish its purpose to relieve the pain in my foot, and for months it was actually worse. One year after this surgery, I was still wearing shoes without backs and limping. Gradually, the swelling did decrease, but to this day I have a lump on my heel, limiting my choice of shoes. The two-inch scar reminds me of the ordeal that accompanied my foot surgery, and the resolve to leave my left foot alone.

Exactly one week after surgery on my right foot, I was meeting my thyroid surgeon. After examining my records, he snapped at me about waiting so long to take care of the thyroid condition, stating that fifty percent of cases like mine were cancerous. I calmly let him know that my oncologist was aware of the spot found on my first PET scan, but was addressing the more pressing matter of breast cancer first. He seemed satisfied with that answer, softening his demeanor.

Discussing a date for surgery caused him to bristle again as I expressed my desire to wait until Spring break in March, avoiding the Christmas holidays as well as missing more school. He definitely wasn't a fan of waiting that long so we settled on two days before Thanksgiving, making it the second surgery I would be having within six weeks.

Again, I was using my valuable holiday time to recuperate from surgery. Anyone who is a teacher understands how important vacations are. A teacher works hard during the school year planning lessons, evaluating, grading, creating, and of course teaching. The well-earned holidays are cherished. I didn't have holidays to speak of during the year of my chemo treatments and, so far this year, I would be giving up additional holidays for surgery. On the other hand, I considered this a better choice than missing days of school.

Like the foot surgery, I was quiet about my thyroid surgery. I didn't want the fuss or attention, or others thinking I might still be dealing with cancer.

The interesting thing about the thyroid nodule was that if it was cancer, I may not have found out for years if I hadn't had breast cancer. The spot was discovered during my first PET scan. If it wasn't cancer, then this would be a pointless surgery, brought on by information discovered because of the breast cancer. As much as I didn't want my thyroid to be cancerous, I also didn't want to lose it unnecessarily. I was tempted to wait until more time had passed and I could see if there were any changes. Remembering the urgency in the thyroid surgeon's voice caused me to contemplate my options carefully. After much consideration, I felt best about going ahead with the surgery, placing my trust in the specialist I had hired.

Thyroid surgery is a relatively simple procedure. I woke up with little pain and only expected to stay overnight in the hospital. The whole thing would have been without incident, except the bleeding at the site of my incision wouldn't stop. The nurses tried everything they knew, but blood quickly soaked up all the dressings they placed. I heard them put calls in for the doctor without receiving a response, and I listened as they conferred in the hallway about what to try next. Two of my friends had stopped by to visit, but they were finally asked to leave so full attention could be addressed to the problem. I remained relatively calm throughout the evening, but was relieved when the surgeon finally did return the calls and told the nurse to simply apply direct pressure. I think the nurse was hesitant to do that on a fresh incision, which is why she didn't try it earlier. After applying direct pressure for about fifteen minutes, the bleeding finally stopped and I was left alone to sleep for the night.

When the surgeon returned the following morning to check on me, he was somewhat apologetic about the bleeding incident the night before. I could tell by his demeanor and comments he was irritated at the nurses, but I didn't complain and made light of the incident. As far as I could see, the problem was that he wasn't answering his phone, causing the real delay.

All I cared about was that I was free to go home, with instructions on how to care for the incision and to call the office for a return visit. Thankfully, recovery was without further incident. The day after Thanksgiving I received a call from my surgeon with the good news that the tumor was not cancer. I was relieved by the news, but couldn't help but think I had endured an unnecessary procedure which resulted in having to take thyroid medicine the rest of my life.

After my foot and thyroid surgery, life finally settled down. My physical challenges resulting from two surgeries paled in comparison to the previous year of chemo treatments. Due to my daily contact with sweet children, I was gradually healing emotionally. I began to see some progress in recovery as I stepped further and further away from my cancer diagnosis.

I was now on a schedule for seeing Dr. Polowy every three months and my next appointment was in March. One week before each visit, I would go to the Cancer Center to have my port flushed and blood drawn. I always entered the clinic with some degree of trepidation, wary of the familiar antiseptic smell that always brought back so many memories. Sometimes I would feel strong and could stand up to the wave of feelings that consumed me. Other times I felt small and powerless against the flood of emotions.

On that spring day in March, I walked in confidently, feeling somewhat removed for the first time from the label of cancer patient. When my name was called and I walked into the chemo room, I was thrilled to see several nurses I knew. We exchanged hugs as I expressed joy in seeing these women who had skillfully performed their job as well as being a comfort during my many hours of treatment.

One of the nurses asked how long it had been since my last chemo which made me realize that I was almost one year out. How grateful I was to be feeling more like myself again. As I sat there waiting for Debbie to flush my port, tears began rolling down my face. Here I was, healthy and finally well, remembering how many times I sat in that very room receiving chemotherapy or hydration. Around me were others who sat where I once was, patiently waiting for their IV bags to drain. My tears were a mixture of empathy for these patients and gratitude for my progress. It was a time to count my blessings and my heart swelled with emotion for the journey and lessons learned.

The next week was my three-month checkup with Dr. Polowy. I looked forward to this time when I could ask questions and receive reassurance that all continued to be well. He was always patient and never seemed in a hurry during my appointments. I remember back to the time when I was contemplating which oncologist to choose. How grateful I was that I had chosen well.

When Dr. Polowy walked in he exclaimed with genuine enthusiasm how great I was looking. Of course, compared to my very worst chemo day, anything was an improvement. My only concern at this appointment was the continuing problem of sleepless nights due to anxiety. He reassured me that it was fine to keep taking the medicine he prescribed to help me relax at night and get a good rest.

As he went through his usual routine, checking for lumps or anything suspicious, we casually chatted. Dr. Polowy said he was going to send a report to Dr. Deyden about my excellent progress. The best news was that it was time to take out my port. Removing the port was a huge step in regaining confidence in my health. I had finally arrived at the point where even my oncologist felt I had licked cancer. As excited as I was to have this apparatus gone, there was a part of me that held back. I wasn't absolutely convinced that a cancer cell wasn't still present, lurking silently, hiding, waiting to present itself again when least expected. What was it going to take to trust again? How long before I could shake off this fear?

When my appointment had ended, I was grateful with my progress over the year and that I had finally arrived at a place where cancer didn't consume my every thought. I was on the road to recovery and significant growth had been made, but there were still a few lurking foes I had to conquer.

*August 24, 2012*

*Dear Journal,*

*I'm torn in every direction. First of all, I am an advocate for modern medicine. Believe me, I have heard plenty of miracle cures from well-meaning acquaintances—anything from taking four tablespoons of canned creamed asparagus a day (someone left an article about that on my doorstep) to health supplements sold by individuals in a multi-level marketing company. I respect their opinions, but I believe in the results of years of scientific research.*

*That is why it is so difficult for me to not comply with the hormone therapy Dr. Polowy prescribed. I know it is the right choice to help prevent a recurrence, but it makes me feel horrible.*

*The Danish philosopher Soren Kierkegaard summed up my dilemma well. "I see it all perfectly; there are two possible situations—one can either do this or that. My honest opinion and my friendly advice is this: do it or do not do it—you will regret both."*

11

# THE TROUBLE WITH DRUGS

The two major post-chemo obstacles I struggled with were, first, the fear of cancer returning and, second, living with the drug designed to prevent my cancer from returning. I recognized I could diminish the size of the first obstacle—fear—by simply taking the drug my oncologist prescribed. Such a solution appeared logical, but it was not as easy as it seemed.

Cancer patients are informed about the importance of hormone therapy which is generally given after chemotherapy to those with hormone receptor positive breast cancer. The recommended duration is for five years, but recently this has been extended to ten years for some patients. I had been taught at my first appointment the benefits of combined therapy which included chemotherapy followed by hormone therapy, and I agreed to that regimen.

Having successfully completed chemo, I felt I had reached home plate. The rest was easy. Dr. Polowy prescribed Arimidex, the hormone drug given to post-menopausal patients, and I never doubted my ability to continue with the next phase of treatment.

Arimidex can cause bone loss and so I had a bone density scan to determine my baseline before beginning this drug. A bone density scan is quick and simple and should not be confused with a bone scan that is used to diagnose abnormalities of the bone such as cancer. Since the scan was favorable, I began taking Arimidex in June, three months after my last chemo. In the beginning, I tolerated it very well. When I visited Dr. Polowy after taking it for a few months, I told him about pain I was having in my feet and knees. He assured me that was one of the side effects of Arimidex and it was quite acceptable to take an anti-inflammatory to help relieve the aching. Dr. Polowy appreciated my efforts to stick with this drug, indicating there were some who gave up. He reiterated the importance of Arimidex in decreasing the odds of cancer metastasizing.

The longer I took Arimidex however, the more I noticed increasing problems associated with this medicine. By September, I was beginning to feel like an old lady. I needed assistance to stand, and my knees didn't like climbing or descending stairs. Even my jaw ached and would crack when I chewed. The bones in my elbows hurt to be touched. Arimidex, designed to be my advocate, was becoming my enemy.

In October, I went to the Cancer Center for a scheduled port flush and decided to mention these symptoms to the oncology nurse. She must have thought my complaint was legitimate enough to personally relay my discomfort to Dr. Polowy. When she came back to report his recommendations, I was surprised to hear he had ordered a bone scan. I knew what he was thinking. The pain I was having could mean the cancer had spread to my bones. She also relayed the doctor's orders to stop taking Arimidex for a few months.

Trying to fit a bone scan appointment into the week before Fall break was tricky. I was also preparing for foot surgery the next week and needed every available minute to get things ready to complete first quarter report cards. Dr. Polowy wanted the scan before surgery and so two days later, I was at the imaging center. This would be my second bone scan, the first one occurring in the hospital after my mastectomy. This subsequent check was far more detailed and lengthy than the first scan. In all, it probably took a good forty-five minutes.

When the scan was complete, along with a few X-rays of the most painful areas, the technician showed me some of the films, but I couldn't tell if anything unusual was found. I would just have to be patient and wait for the results.

Even though I was anxious to hear the outcome of my scan, the next few days were so busy I didn't have time to indulge in much worry. At the end of the week, I called Dr. Polowy's office to get the results. I received my return call within a few hours with the good news that breast cancer hadn't invaded my bones. Arimidex was to blame for my discomfort, which was a far better scenario than stage four cancer.

I decided to stay off the Arimidex until my next appointment with Dr. Polowy, at which time I would discuss my options with him. The joints still ached and continued to do so for at least a month, then gradually diminished. It was a relief to be able to bend my elbows without pain. My knees felt better, but I still stood slowly and it took a few minutes to loosen up. Even though the side effects were fading, I wondered if I would be able to take the Arimidex again. No matter what I decided, there would be consequences for either choice.

In December of 2010, I met with Dr. Polowy for my three-month appointment. I was feeling better and with the memory of previous joint pain fading, I decided to tackle the Arimidex again. He supported me with enthusiasm and I must admit I felt better about making the effort to do all I could to comply with the recommended therapy. The Arimidex was the main topic of discussion during this visit as everything else was going well.

At my next visit in March, I could report continued success with Arimidex. I had taken it for three months and so far, I hadn't noticed any complications or the side effects I had previously experienced. Both Dr. Polowy and I were encouraged and I was proud of myself for being able to stick with the program.

Around the following June, I noticed the same bone and joint pain I had experienced previously, creeping back to annoy me. I decided to dig in my heels and try and tolerate what was pretty reliable insurance against breast cancer returning. I think I would have been successful with this resolve if things had remained constant.

As time went on, the pain kept escalating, making it difficult to do simple things such as stand up from a sitting position, or lift my arms to comb my hair. If I were to get down on the floor, I couldn't get up without assistance. Dr. Polowy prescribed a mild pain reliever, Tramadol, designed for chronic pain, and encouraged me to stick with the Arimidex. He was hopeful I wouldn't give up, and I was determined to endure. I kept thinking how difficult chemotherapy had been and if I could get through that, I surely could stick with the other half of the formula.

At first I was reluctant to take Tramadol. The last thing I wanted was to become dependent on pain medication. In the past, I was careful to take minimal doses of any pain medicine I was prescribed, even after a surgery, often preferring pain over how the medicine made me feel. I filled the prescription but only took it when I couldn't stand the aching any longer. In the beginning, that amounted to about twice a week. As the pain increased, I gave in and took it once a day, choosing when I needed it the most, during my hours at school. It didn't take long to notice that I felt pretty good when I was on the medicine, so I finally gave up the fight and took it regularly, as prescribed, which was every twelve hours.

During this time, I felt like I could function normally again. I still experienced minor joint aches, but I could walk and move comfortably. I also felt more energy and zest for life. Having energy was extremely important in my job as a teacher. Encouraged that I had figured out a solution I could live with, I eagerly embraced my responsibilities, relishing in the ability to reclaim my life.

Unfortunately, the relief didn't last more than a few months. The pain began to increase at the same time the efficacy of the pain medicine began to decrease. It seemed apparent that in order to alleviate this, I would have to keep increasing the amount of pain medicine and that's where I drew the line. I didn't want to live the next five years escalating the doses of pain medication to counter the intensified side effects caused by Arimidex, and I knew I had to make a decision.

Words can't describe the inward battle I waged during these months of trial and error. Knowledge of the benefits of hormone therapy warred with my body's intolerance of it. Quality of life was being compromised, yet I wanted to embrace the recommended path to eradicate cancer. It wasn't an easy decision and I was influenced by outside voices; voices of people who cared about me. My children didn't want me to give up on the Arimidex, concerned about the consequences. Randy was an everyday witness of the painful limitations of the drug, but knew how important its role was in completing my treatment for cancer. My son, now a medical student, encouraged me to follow my doctor's advice. In an effort to help in my dilemma and provide another avenue for treatment, Dr. Polowy prescribed Tamoxifen, an alternate hormone drug. No longer trusting medicine, I put the prescription in my drawer where it stayed untouched for six months.

In the meantime, I was dealing with a great deal of pain in my arms and legs. I stopped taking the Arimidex the first week of December and hoped that by Christmas I would be feeling myself again. Gradually, the aching subsided to where the pain medicine, which I continued to take, resumed working. I was not anxious to start Tamoxifen until the side effects of the Arimidex had vanished. I didn't realize how long I would have to wait for that to occur.

At my next visit with Dr. Polowy, I had to confess that I hadn't started the Tamoxifen yet. He was concerned with the constant pain I was still experiencing as he had never seen the side effects of Arimidex go beyond three months. I'm sure he was also concerned that I was not taking any of the drugs designed to help prevent cancer from reoccurring. He ordered more blood tests to make sure other factors were not contributing to my symptoms.

When all the tests came back negative, we could only conclude I was still experiencing the damage Arimidex had done to my body. Despite his desire that I stick with the prescribed five-year plan for hormone therapy, Dr. Polowy was never pushy. He respected my feelings and even though he preferred that I follow what years of research had proven, he listened and counseled with compassion, offering support for the decision only I could make. Sharing that there were others who struggled with these drugs helped me not feel so alone and isolated in my dilemma.

It all came down to trust. I had trusted the Arimidex and now I was paying for it. I had to weigh the prospects of starting something new, with similar warnings of possible side effects, or take a chance on cancer returning. To a bystander, the right choice appears obvious. For me, the decision seemed ominous as I was dealing with constant pain, which necessitated reliance on pain medication. This brought with it the potential for addiction, an unexpected cancer effect I did not want to experience.

I found myself making excuses for my lack of compliance. I pulled out the paper with the original bar graph I had saved since my initial visit with Dr. Polowy. The chances of cancer returning were only 23% higher if I didn't take the prescribed hormone receptor drug for five years. I did take it for nearly one year, off and on, which had to be somewhat beneficial.

Every time I thought of trying Tamoxifen, fear of the possible side effects pushed the thought aside. Once I actually took the prescription out of my drawer to fill it. Stapled to the prescription were two pages that explained the drug and its possible side effects. After carefully reading them, I put all three pages back in my drawer. I wasn't ready to take a chance, especially when I was finally feeling better.

What would this delay mean in the long run? How would I feel if my cancer did metastasize and how would I explain that to my family, especially my grandchildren? Was I ready to suffer through another round of treatment for cancer? To make matters worse, one of my friends lost her battle with cancer during this time of mental turmoil. All these conflicting factors caused a lot of anxiety when I wanted to be celebrating two years of being cancer free.

Fresh on my mind was a recent encounter with a cancer patient named Marge. I met her at the first breast cancer support group meeting I attended. She was young with children living at home and like me, was still wearing her wig, indicating that the memory of chemo was fresh. In her introductions at the meeting, she confessed that she stopped taking Tamoxifen, the hormone receptor drug she had been prescribed. She merely stated that the side effects were more than she could handle, and that her "children and husband were done". Those were her exact words, and I could certainly relate to her sentiment now that I was struggling with the same problem.

Several months later I was in the Cancer Center waiting to have my port flushed. I looked up to see Marge coming into the waiting room from the doctors' offices. As she solemnly sat, I was tempted to introduce myself again and visit while waiting to enter the infusion room. Since I didn't really know her, and she seemed deep in thought, I hesitated. We were both called into the infusion room about the same time and I watched as the nurses started an IV and attached a large bag filled with a chemo drug to the pole by her chair.

The scene impacted me deeply. I was standing at the crossroads myself, trying to decide if I should resume hormonal therapy. Would I be in her shoes someday because

I decided to stop the recommended treatment? Was this chance encounter meant to teach me a lesson? I was never able to erase this scene from my mind during the months I agonized over which direction I should take. Watching Marge begin chemo again would be a nagging reminder of what could happen.

Another summer came, and a vacation from my teaching responsibilities and structured routine. I was determined to use this time to make some important decisions about the Tamoxifen. It was time to take the prescription out of my drawer and give it a try. I owed it to myself, my family, and my doctor to make an effort, and there was no better time than summer when I could afford to experiment.

It had now been close to seven months since I had gone off the Arimidex; seven months without taking the prescribed hormone therapy for my breast cancer. I was treading dangerous water. With determination, I clutched the prescription, climbed into my car and drove the two blocks to the pharmacy. Proud of my audacity to accomplish something I had dreaded for so long, I plopped the filled bottle on my bathroom counter, in full sight. Filling the prescription was one thing. Taking it was another.

As each day passed and I didn't open the bottle, I finally put it away, hoping to silence the nagging. The Tamoxifen stayed in my medicine cabinet for a full month before I finally talked myself into trying it. I would set a date to start, and then find what I thought were good reasons to wait until another day. I did a lot of self-reflection during this time, trying to determine what was keeping me from moving forward. I knew the principle obstacle was fear—fear that my feeling of wellness would disappear when I took the Tamoxifen with its long list of possible side effects. But what about the fear of cancer returning? That was certainly a deeply imbedded fear. I needed to make a decision.

Finally, two weeks before I was to meet with Dr. Polowy for my three-month check-up, I took my first Tamoxifen.

Probably my biggest motivator at the time was that I wanted to tell him that I made the correct choice to begin, even if it was just recently. Two weeks into a drug is not an indicator of its potential for problems but Dr. Polowy was pleased with my decision to start, and happy that I had no side effects to report. I'm not sure if he knew I had only started recently. I think he was just happy I started.

By the time I saw my oncologist in the fall, I had to report that I didn't stick with the Tamoxifen. In fact, I never refilled the prescription, meaning that I took this drug for 30 days and decided the side effects weren't worth it. The aching was beginning to return, but I also had additional problems with discharge and hot flashes. My tolerance for medicinal side effects by now was zero and so rather than stick it out, I just stopped. Like Marge, I was done. I decided to keep this decision to myself. If my family thought I was following the recommended path, they wouldn't worry. My husband, and eventually Dr. Polowy were the only ones who knew I had made my final decision to quit hormonal therapy.

As difficult as the choice was, I feel it was right for me. What is right for me isn't necessarily right for others. Each breast cancer patient needs to make her own decision concerning the five-year hormonal therapy. Many are very successful and I not only applaud them, I envy them. How I wish I could have found success in completing the recommended treatment plan. An internal tug-of-war waged as I weighed the quality of my life against the chances of shortening my life, but once the decision was made, I tried not to look back. Any lack of confidence in my resolution was overshadowed by the fact that I was finally feeling better. Being active, achieving as much as possible each day, and enjoying my family were so important to me that I couldn't envision living the rest of my life lacking energy and physical well-being.

Having made the decision to not comply with the hormone therapy, I discovered my battle with drugs was far from over. The side-effects from the Arimidex had long worn off but I was still taking Tramadol twice a day. I wanted to eliminate it, but my body had become accustomed to the constant supply I provided, and I felt sick if I missed a dose. On one occasion, I had left home to run some errands and had forgotten to take my morning pill. Not having any with me, I turned the car around and returned home. From experience, I knew how I would feel if I didn't take the medicine on time. This was just one example of how Tramadol ruled my life. I was living proof of what I feared would occur when I started taking this drug. Finding myself a slave to its power over me, I wasn't sure when and how I could escape.

I needed to function at my best while teaching school, so I continued taking the Tramadol regularly for nearly three years. I knew the time would come when it would be necessary to eliminate this drug and I voiced my concerns to my primary care physician. He admitted it would be "ugly", but suggested I quit "cold turkey". I voiced my concerns to Dr. Polowy and he referred me to a pain specialist who had the knowledge and training to help overcome dependence on medications.

The pain specialist was understanding and compassionate of my situation. Since I was on such a low dosage of Tramadol, he thought I could handle the situation myself by just cutting each pill in half and lengthening the time between doses. My appointment with him was helpful as he gave me the confidence I needed to start. He acknowledged I would feel uncomfortable for a few days, but encouraged me to stick with my resolve. Assuring me it should take less than a week or two to conquer my dependency on Tramadol, I left his office feeling I had the tools necessary to eliminate it from my life.

School had ended and I was in my first week of vacation. I had a few commitments already, but that would be true of the entire summer. It would be best to begin right away with my decision to quit taking Tramadol and have the remainder of the summer to enjoy. I started on a Wednesday morning, cutting a Tramadol pill in half. The first day went well until late afternoon. My body suddenly recognized that it didn't get enough of what it thought it needed. I tried to busy myself to keep my mind off the discomfort. I lacked energy to do anything which was probably the most annoying symptom so far.

The first night was difficult. Not only was my sleep continually interrupted, I ached all over and was jittery. The volume on the buzzing in my ears was turned up several notches. During this sleeplessness, I gave myself pep talks about the importance of not giving in. How I wanted to grab the bottle and take just one more pill so I could feel better. I resisted, knowing such action would set me back and I would have to start again. My goal was to be done with this mess in three to four days. I could hardly wait to flush the remainder of my prescription down the toilet.

The next morning, I anxiously took my half dose but found I only felt worse. Half was virtually the same as taking nothing on the second day, and by evening I determined that the sooner I could completely rid myself of this dependency, the better. I didn't want to have this sick feeling longer than necessary so I decided not to take a half dose at bedtime. That was it. I vowed I would never put a Tramadol in my mouth again. I find it interesting that I still didn't throw the rest of my prescription away after making this promise. Despite my determination, there was a small thread of doubt that kept a few pills available, just in case.

I was now at war with my body. My spirit struggled to be strong and stick to my plan, but my body was in rebellion with nausea, sweats, body aches, and no energy. At night when I would try to escape the sick feeling, I couldn't sleep due to restless leg syndrome and insomnia. When I did drift off from pure exhaustion, I would have crazy vivid dreams, only to wake up and remain awake for hours.

Throughout all of this, I still had things to do. Even though I wasn't teaching school, I had appointments, events to attend, and regular day to day responsibilities. After being without the Tramadol for over 48 hours I had to help a friend with her daughter's wedding reception, assisting in food preparation several hours prior to the celebration. I had volunteered a month ago and when I make a commitment I feel I have to follow through. I showed up, determined to act as normal as possible so as not reveal how badly I was feeling. It reminded me of the days I had to appear at school and teach after a chemo treatment. One thing I have learned from this whole experience is self-discipline. Sometimes you just do what you are required to do. When my assignment was finally finished, I went home, exhausted not only from the physical work, but from having to act like nothing was amiss. I wasn't proud of my dependency, although it wasn't my fault. I took the medicine in good faith and Dr. Polowy prescribed it to help me feel better. Neither of us expected that a small dose would cause such dependence.

Finally, four days after quitting, I started to feel like I was getting my body back. I had turned the corner. With confidence, I decisively flushed the remainder of the prescription away. That step alone was huge. By getting rid of any trace of Tramadol, I had reached my goal, I had won the fight.

Two good things came from this experience. First, I gained an understanding of how difficult it is to overcome an addiction, whether it is to food, drugs, alcohol, or a bad habit. It takes a lot of strength to stick with it, knowing how much easier it is to ignore the problem instead of facing it. I have compassion for others who struggle with habits they wish to eliminate. The road is thorny and grueling, and I don't fault anyone for not making it on a first attempt.

Second, I was finally free—free of pain medicine I habitually took for almost three years. When I felt I hadn't accomplished much my first week of summer vacation, I would be reminded that I achieved mastery over myself. I had been successful in tossing the crutch that was no longer needed. By the end of that summer, three years since my final chemo treatment, I was finally feeling close to my original self. I had whittled my medicinal intake to thyroid medicine and had resolved the inner turmoil over the hormone therapy. Unknown were the consequences of that decision, but mentally, I had achieved some peace, and physically, I had overcome my dependency on Tramadol. When I began chemotherapy, I never expected to face a battle with drugs. I was the victim to one, but the victor over the other. I have grown from both conflicts.

*October 13, 2011*

*Dear Journal,*

*This evening at our support group meeting one of the breast cancer survivors stated, "No one can take away your femininity."*

*Maybe mentally, but physically it certainly has been compromised.*

12

# INSTEAD, I HAVE CURLS

Cancer compromises whatever body part it chooses to invade. For the breast cancer patient, to preserve our lives, we must often surrender that which is a hallmark of our femininity. When cancer was discovered, I wanted all traces removed quickly and completely, and in my case, a bilateral mastectomy was required. Hearing the surgeon's recommendations, I consented, grateful for any chance to prolong my life.

There is no way to prepare for the repercussions of losing one or both breasts. Most breast cancer victims don't begin the process of mourning their loss until months, even years later. The patient is focused on eradicating the cancer and surviving treatment. When that is complete, she looks down, finally facing the full realization that she sacrificed her breasts in the process.

This is one of the most profound effects of breast cancer and it impacted my life more than I wanted to acknowledge or confront. As the years have passed since losing my breasts, I haven't adjusted to their absence, nor has it become easier to accept. I am reminded every day they are gone.

I can still remember my early teens, those delightful years when a girl begins to develop breasts. The minor growing pains are superseded by the excitement of leaving childhood to become a young woman. Those around me were in all stages of development, and I was bringing up the rear. It didn't matter because it was happening.

Buying my first bra was a momentous occasion. It was about as tiny as they come. I don't think I weighed more than eighty-five pounds and my new beginnings barely filled the smallest sized cup. With time and patience, I proudly moved forward to a larger bra, but still at the beginning of the alphabet. Then, the growing stopped. Being small busted didn't bother me like it did some girls, and I simply accepted it for what it was. For my frame, they were perfect, and I was satisfied.

There were some perks to being petite. When I was old, I wouldn't sag. It's funny what is important when we are young, and wisdom hasn't yet taught us there could be worse issues than sagging.

Randy fell in love with me, not my breasts, but they were certainly a part of the package. He liked them, too. I'm not the only one who misses them.

After my bilateral mastectomy, I didn't make any effort to explore the available options for replacing my breasts. I did the easiest thing, which was to place two little stuffed forms that I received at the hospital into my existing bra.

I learned very quickly, and the hard way, that they do not like to stay in place. As I was teaching my second-graders one day near the beginning of my treatment, I glanced down to see both stuffed forms had worked their way up and out of my bra for all to see. I immediately turned around towards the white board and stuffed them back in.

After that, I always remembered to pin them down carefully in place. This simple method of breast replacement worked for the first year, and I didn't have any pressing desire to buy mastectomy bras and silicone breast forms. It wasn't an issue of money as my health insurance paid the bill, but it was a matter of mustering up the energy to find a better solution. It would mean being fitted, making choices, and most of all admitting that my breasts were really missing, all of which I couldn't handle in my present emotional state.

After chemo was complete, I decided to check out the possibility of breast reconstruction. Dr. Polowy referred me to a good plastic surgeon, one who was noted for his reconstructive surgery. I was told by Dr. Deyden I needed to wait one full year before having this procedure. That time had nearly arrived, so I made an appointment.

Randy and I took some time to look on-line at various results of breast reconstruction. I wasn't impressed with what I saw. In fact, I was mortified. I don't know what I was expecting, but I didn't anticipate seeing the scar run across unnatural, often lopsided breasts topped with artificial, tattooed nipples. Some pictures looked good, but I wondered about the ones that didn't. What would a person do if their case was one that turned out poorly? I was filled with skepticism when it was time for my appointment.

The plastic surgeon was young and very personable. After examining me he took ample time to explain how he would approach my reconstruction. I would need surgery, which would be a more painful procedure than a mastectomy since muscle would be involved. Following initial surgery during which balloon-like objects would be inserted, the skin would be gradually stretched by periodically inflating the balloons. The surgeon didn't spare the news that this procedure was quite painful.

When a patient achieved the desired size, another surgery would remove the balloons and replace them with the substance chosen. Next would be additional surgery to remove flesh from one part of the body to make nipples, followed by tattooing to achieve a realistic appearance.

Upon hearing the entire procedure, I thanked the doctor and walked out, never planning to return. After going through the last nine months, I was done with doctors, surgeries, and pain. Luckily, my husband supported this decision. I was comfortable with my present circumstances and I felt so blessed that he loved me the way I was. If I ever changed my mind, insurance was required to pay. It was an option I left open, but for the moment I was done with surgical procedures.

I decided to take an alternate route and check with my insurance company on where to go for mastectomy bras and breast prostheses. I had learned from my wig experience that I needed to find places that accepted my insurance if I expected them to cover the cost and I knew those items could be expensive. When I found a company, I made an appointment for a fitting.

I was pleasantly surprised to meet and work with a kind woman who took time to explain my options and provide me with multiple bras to try on. She spent at least a full hour helping me decide on several styles and giving instruction on caring for and using my breast forms. The company checked my insurance benefits, and found they were willing to provide me with six bras a year, and new breast forms every two years. I couldn't imagine owning six bras, having only two at a time when I was required to buy them. I thought it a bit frivolous to own that many at once, but gratefully accepted my good fortune, choosing three different styles for variety. I ended up preferring one style and the next year I purchased six of those.

I adapted to my new bras and breast forms easily and wished I had made that transition soon after my bilateral mastectomy. But then I realized I was moving at my own speed, adjusting to my new body at a rate I could manage. Later, when I changed insurance companies, my benefits expanded to an unlimited number of bras each year. Not only that, I was sent to an elite department store where I could choose from any of their lines of bras, not just bras designed for mastectomy patients. They would send them out and sew pocket linings into each cup, forming a little nest to hold the prostheses in place. This time, I chose from a large selection of colors and styles, making me feel somewhat closer to being normal again. There is something about wearing a bra with a little lace and design that restores a small measure of femininity.

Early on, I found I could hide my deficiency with clothes, as long as I was careful to check and make sure I wasn't lopsided. An outsider probably would never know the difference. But I do. I don't look at myself very often in the mirror. I shy away from Randy looking at me. Physically, I *feel* incomplete.

For breast cancer patients who desire reconstruction, there are several choices when it comes to replacing what cancer took away. Some are fortunate to start the process of reconstruction during the same surgery performed to remove the tumor. This was the case of one of my survivor friends. During her mastectomy, expanders were inserted followed by several weeks of silicone injections to rebuild her breasts to the desired size. Although she would do it again, she admits they don't feel the same as her natural breasts. They are heavier and she is more conscious of their presence, especially when trying to sleep on her stomach. She likes how she looks in her clothes, especially a swimsuit, but looking in the mirror and seeing the scar running across the middle is a constant reminder they are not what they are supposed to be. The lack of sensation or feeling in reconstructed breasts rules out their romantic role and is sorely missed.

Another means of reconstruction that is even more invasive is called the TRAM-flap method. This procedure is preferred by some as it involves one's own tissue rather than a foreign implant. Those who choose this method or one like it are usually patients who were not able to have immediate reconstruction. Such was the case of another friend who waited nearly two years for clearance to begin. She described the procedure of using her abdominal tissues and muscles to rebuild her breasts and the extreme pain she experienced from the resulting surgeries, followed by months of physical therapy. It has been four years since her reconstruction and she continues to experience discomfort. Despite all she went through she declares she would do it again as opposed to being concave when looking in the mirror. Her emotional struggles have a familiar ring with other survivors, as she describes her disappointment in how they look, along with the absence of feeling.

Am I sorry I never opted for reconstructive surgery? Except for some numbness in the surgical area, my skin still has feeling and I'm not burdened with heavy artificial breasts that basically have no purpose but to look good under clothes. In all three examples, which include two types of reconstruction, or no reconstruction, I see very little difference. We are all still missing our breasts.

A common theme among the breast cancer survivors I have met is the dramatic effect that cancer has played with intimacy. Physically, the cancer survivor is not only missing one or both breasts, but she has often been hurried into early menopause. The hormones provided for most women to counter the resulting issues are cancer-causing. Dr. Polowy referred me to a specialist in women's pelvic medicine and surgery to get some help with the dryness I was experiencing and frequent bladder infections. I was very impressed with the specialist's knowledge and he was a huge help in improving my bladder function. When it came to my other issues, he apologetically admitted that he couldn't give me what I needed due to my hormone positive cancer. He did provide me with a cream that was only available at a woman's pharmacy. It was helpful for a while, but soon lost its effectiveness.

Not easily defeated, I listened to ideas from other survivors, given in group meetings on the rare occasions it was discussed. Buying a recommended product, I would excitedly exclaim to Randy that I thought I finally solved the problem. Over and over, we were disappointed. Once I watched a web seminar titled *Intimacy after Cancer*, hopeful for some answers. It was a well-planned presentation, but its approach was broad, offering no real workable solutions. The program concluded acknowledging that yes, the problem existed and the medical explanations for why.

My close survivor friends and I have had more detailed discussions, sharing our frustrations, and any insights we've discovered. We all agree that the lack of normal intimacy causes all kinds of issues and so we struggle to find answers as well as solutions. It is a process we face and it takes time to figure out. Many are fortunate to have understanding husbands to help them get through it. One found that her husband didn't look at her any differently, but that it took her years to come to the realization that she was still a woman, attractive to her husband, and a loving person. Many of us compensate with different ways of showing affection, taking time to make our spouse feel valued and loved. Communication goes a long way in this process along with a huge dose of patience, acceptance, and time.

The subject of intimacy after breast cancer is an elusive one. It is rarely addressed. When it is, it's so vague the patient and her spouse are left to stumble along figuring things out alone. From my experience and those of my close survivor friends, I feel the solution is found within. We all must come to terms with the changes we now face, recognizing and accepting the fact we are still women with the same capacity to love and nurture that we've always had.

Over the last seven years, Randy and I have been challenged with the issue of intimacy. I am grateful for an exceptional husband who has patiently worked with me to help make the best out of an adverse situation. He is selfless, gentle, and kind. Randy is an example of someone who loves unconditionally. He loves me for who I am, not for what I have or don't have, not for what was, but what is. The biggest problem lies with my inability to feel comfortable with my own deficiencies.

Our dilemma, along with the threat of cancer returning, led to a conversation most couples never feel the need to discuss. I was the one that brought up the subject.

"If anything happens to me, I would want you to remarry," I blurted out of the blue one summer day.

Being truthful, Randy admitted, "I have wondered what I would do, being faced with years of loneliness. Then I chide myself for not having faith that everything is going to be fine. When I even consider such an option, I feel like I'm giving up, that my faith is wavering."

"Talking, and even thinking about this is not a lack of faith," I consoled him. "When you buy life insurance, you never expect to use it. You don't make out a will because you think you're going to die. You are just being prepared."

"Well, I don't think I could remarry. It makes everything so complicated. What would I do with all our memories, pictures, souvenirs from vacations? There is evidence of you in every room, in every corner of my mind and heart. And I'm positive our children wouldn't accept someone new."

At that point we had a little discussion about the expected reaction received from each of our six children. We laughed at who would tolerate another woman in their dad's life, and who absolutely would not.

Getting back on track with the purpose of the conversation, I continued, "Without a woman around, I'm worried you would live on a diet of fast-food and scrambled egg sandwiches. You would be so lonely, and you absolutely deserve a whole woman again. I have not been that for you these last few years."

"I still don't think it would be worth it. If I'm lonely, I'll get a dog." I could tell Randy didn't want to discuss the matter any longer.

I summed it up where I began, just to be certain he knew where I stood. "I want to make sure you know it would be okay if you decide to remarry if I die." To lighten the mood, I added, "As long as she's not good looking or well endowed."

The undeniable fact is that life isn't the same after breast cancer and the survivor must make whatever adjustments she can to function with the cards she has been dealt. When my hair grew in curly, I felt that physically I had received a small degree of compensation. It was a personal gift designed for me, as I always equated curls with femininity. Still sporting those curls, I treasure the meaning they have for me. Breast cancer robbed me of my breasts and many of my natural feminine feelings. The curls helped restore some of my losses, if only mentally.

Curls can never replace my breasts but since there is nothing I can do to get them back, I accept what I can't change and move on.

*October 16, 2011*

*Dear Journal,*

*Can you smell the fresh, clean, pine-filled scent of Fall in the mountains? I just came back from fly fishing with a volunteer from Casting for Recovery. He was an experienced fisherman, and my buddy and mentor as I applied all I had learned these last few days.*

*We caught one small trout, and as exciting as that was, it didn't come close to the conversation I had with him. His mom had just been diagnosed with breast cancer and he asked for advice on how he could best help her.*

*The opportunity to give back was the most fulfilling of these incredible three days in the pines. It has been a long time since I've experienced so much joy and peace. I don't want to leave this place, or the friends I've made.*

*Most importantly, I have discovered that healing is accomplished through serving others.*

13

# HELP IN HEALING

With cancer, there are several layers of healing. The most obvious layer is the physical and it lies in the hands of the oncologist. Less recognized are the emotional, mental, and social layers. These layers are most often set aside until physical healing is complete at which time they surface and demand attention. I was oblivious to the many options available to help cancer patients obtain full recovery and the helping hands extended to lift and support. They were out there, but first I had to recognize I needed help, and then make the effort to discover and embrace all they had to offer.

As I became more acquainted with the programs offered at my cancer center and other venues, I was amazed that there were so many organizations and volunteers available for those facing cancer, and for those recovering and trying to put their lives back together. As I participated in these groups, I developed a whole network of new friends and still enjoy my association with these amazing people.

Every year the hospital hosts "A Cancer Survivor's Celebration". It happened to occur right after my chemo was completed and I was going through some rough emotional times. When I received the invitation, I decided to attend. It was my first attempt to finally take the steps to help myself and meet other survivors. I was really looking forward to this celebration that featured a motivational speaker who was also a cancer survivor. Luckily the date fell in the beginning of the summer so I didn't have a conflict with my teaching job.

On the day of the celebration, I decided not to take my cell phone or wear a watch. I didn't want to be interrupted or worry about time. It was truly a day to get away and be with other people whose lives had been touched by cancer. This was a new experience for me, but the beginning of many more opportunities to be buoyed up as stories and feelings were shared. I can't stress how much it helped to know the emotions that ran rampant through me were felt by others as well.

As I walked in, I was greeted by two therapy dogs, brought by the hospital staff to the celebration. Petting them, I was reminded of the important role dogs play in helping cancer patients. My golden retriever, Sunny, was a good companion during the days following each chemo treatment. He knew I wasn't myself and would lay by me for hours, occasionally licking my hands or legs. Many times, we were the only two at home and he would faithfully stay by my side, keeping me company.

I was led to a seat, and because I was by myself, I ended up at the very front, filling in a single space at a table right beneath the podium. At each place setting there was a decorated bag full of various snacks such as granola bars, trail mix, an orange and some candy. There was also a packet for each attendee along with a notebook, pen, and a DVD full of cancer resources. It all looked festive and inviting. I was impressed with the amount of work and detail that went into planning and making sure each survivor felt special and celebrated.

I sat down at a table of complete strangers, but noticed how quickly we all engaged in conversation. It was not really surprising since we shared a common bond. We didn't have much time to visit before a man welcomed us and then introduced Patricia, the hospital oncology counselor. Her friendly manner helped us all feel welcome as she introduced the "Singing Survivors" who had prepared an introductory program for us. They were comprised of about fifteen volunteers who were cancer survivors, hospital staff, or caretakers. For such a small group, they were remarkable.

The first song they sang was *Raindrops Keep Falling on My Head* which I had heard many times through the years. My recent experiences gave new meaning to the words, *"But there's one thing I know, the blues they send to meet me won't defeat me. It won't be long till happiness steps up to greet me."*

The lyrics hit home and tears streamed down my face. Since I was out in front, it was rather embarrassing to be five minutes into this celebration with my emotions already out of control. As the group sang other cheerful songs, I smiled at their enthusiasm and clever choreography. Their signature song, however, brought the tears back as they sang *Lean on Me*. They asked us to stand and join with them, but I was too choked up to sing. As I stood and cried, I was reminded how music can motivate, lift, and inspire. During my months of treatments, music had softened the burden, given me hope, and had encouraged me to move forward. Like a friend, it was always available and could transform any mood into something better.

As the guest speaker was introduced, I was surprised to see her come on stage in a wheelchair. We learned that cancer wasn't her only trial. She was paralyzed from the waist down due to being a victim of a rape and beating while attending college. After being run over by a car and left for dead, she was rescued and treated, fighting with all she had for her life. Recovering as much as possible from this physical and emotional trial, she then found out she had ovarian cancer and enlisted in a new fight for life. As she shared her story with us, I was deeply touched by her strength, courage, and optimism. What an amazing example for all of us in attendance. I came away feeling a whole lot better about my own simple battle, fortified by her tender, courageous words.

After the speaker concluded and cake was served, people began to mingle again and one of the ladies in the support group I attended earlier in the week came up and gave me a hug. It meant so much that she even recognized me. We visited, shared, laughed, and cried together, forming a bond based on empathy for what each had endured. I was making friends with people I never would have had the chance to meet before cancer. I remember my friend Cindy saying I would encounter many amazing people along the way, and her words were being fulfilled. Some I would come across only once, while others became friends in a new fight. Each one brought sunshine, new insights, and a large dose of healing.

One of the best things I did after my chemo treatments ended was attend a breast cancer support group. I didn't do this until summer and was reluctant at first, assuming it was for patients still undergoing treatment. Patricia conducted these meetings and during a phone conversation, explained the gatherings were for everyone in any stage of treatment or survival. I decided to try it out. The group met the fourth Tuesday evening of every month in the radiation waiting room at the hospital.

The first time I attended, I arrived five minutes late since I had trouble locating the meeting area. Already seated in a circle were about ten women of different ages. I quietly slipped into an empty chair and listened as Patricia announced what we would discuss that evening. She asked that we first introduce ourselves and then share our story and one thing that helped us during our cancer journey. A middle-aged woman named Nancy began, and as each participant shared,

I sat spellbound. One thing I've noticed about cancer survivors is that they like to share their stories. I could see why when it was my turn to talk. There was healing in sharing, and by the end of the evening I was overwhelmed with gratitude for the ninety minutes I had taken to give and learn from others. The atmosphere was casual and everyone felt comfortable enough to interject comments or ask questions. Each individual story was unique, but I had never been surrounded by so many women who experienced the feelings and emotions that mirrored mine. We all shared a common bond that began with the words, "You have cancer".

Besides sharing feelings, I gained a lot of valuable information about lymphedema and what to look for as well as ways to try and avoid it. I was surprised to find that more than half of the women in the group that night were wearing compression devices. I remember receiving material about lymphedema in the paper work I received from the Cancer Center. Precautions listed to help prevent this uncomfortable condition included avoiding sunburn, excess heat such as hot tubs, cuts, or weight gain. Blood pressure readings as well as blood draws and IV's were not to be performed on the arm where lymph nodes had been removed. Some survivors struggled with the problem while others were able to avoid it. There didn't seem to be any logical explanation as to why lymphedema skipped around, choosing its victims.

The compression device is a tight skin-colored stretchy material that covers the length of the affected arm, designed to reduce the swelling. Fortunately, I hadn't faced that problem, but was informed that it was good to have one on hand and could be obtained with a prescription from my oncologist. If for no other reason, I would need to wear one when traveling by plane, as the change in air pressure caused swelling and could lead to the development of lymphedema. I had tickets to fly to Utah later that summer and was grateful for the advice.

As the evening ended, I came away renewed and educated. I had left my home searching for help and found it among a diverse group of women who were traveling the same road as I. Over the years I have attended several of these support meetings as time allowed. No two gatherings were alike or frequented by the same people, allowing many opportunities to make new friends, learn from others, and share nuggets of wisdom gained from my own journey. It allowed me to keep my struggles in perspective as I saw the difficult path others tread.

In our state, the American Cancer Society holds a fundraiser every October, aptly named the "Making Strides Against Breast Cancer" walk. During the year I was being treated, my friends and family formed a group in my honor. I attended the event, but waited in the park as they walked the three-mile course, all wearing matching T-shirts.

I saw breast cancer survivors who were wearing commemorative shirts and sashes proudly celebrate as they started off on the walk. I was impressed with their energy and enthusiasm. I could hardly wait for next year when I could join the group of survivors, rejoicing in a battle won.

As the next year approached, I didn't get to participate due to the foot surgery I had the previous month. There was too much going on at the time to even think about the walk. However, the following year I volunteered to be the leader of our support group, organizing and raising money for the Making Strides Against Breast Cancer walk. It was a time of healing for me as I worked to pull together our little group and our families for such a worthy and meaningful cause.

The morning of the walk was exhilarating as we gathered at a meeting place for pictures. We had our own group shirts which read, "I'm Living Proof" while our families and friends wore "Friends of Banner Desert Cancer Center". Kimberly, Brittany, and Julie came to support the walk along with my husband and six of my grandchildren. It was a memorable occasion and I couldn't help but ponder how far I had come in the last two years. So much had happened, and now I was finally the energetic survivor I had always pictured.

Another big help in my path to recovery was "Face in the Mirror". I first came in contact with this organization in the hospital after my bilateral mastectomy. A representative had entered my room the day after surgery and offered to give me a facial and massage my hands and feet. I was surprised at the offer, but too curious to turn her away. She began by gently cleansing my face, using soft, warm towels to rinse and wipe my face clean. The volunteer then asked if I preferred warm or cool colors which helped her choose the shades of eye shadow to apply. She continued to bring out my eyes with her expert application of mascara. Next she spread a small amount of foundation over my face, adding a subtle shade of blush to my cheekbones. Before beginning my massage, she offered me a mirror to view the results.

I actually felt beautiful. Here I sat in a hospital bed recovering from losing my breasts to cancer while this woman performed miracles. She continued by gently massaging my hands and feet with a cream, visiting and learning my story. It was easy to share the feelings of my heart with this genuine, loving stranger. I could tell she enjoyed the time she spent to brighten my day. Her gentle, loving service communicated a desire to help make my cancer journey hopeful. When she was finished, I not only looked but felt better.

As I expressed my gratitude for her time and services, she gathered all the products she had used and placed them in a white cloth bag decorated with an embroidered pink carnation. When she handed me the bulging bag to keep, I was overwhelmed by her generosity and kindness. I wanted to know more about this organization and its mission to bring a different kind of healing at such a critical time.

After my chemo treatments had ended, I received an invitation to attend the grand opening of "Face in the Mirror" at my hospital. The organization had transformed a small room into a beautifully decorated space in which cancer patients could come and receive facials, massages, and pampering. I was desperately in need of a boost and the encouragement I knew this organization could provide. I readily signed up, excited to participate again in this generous outpouring of support for cancer patients. Surgery to remove both breasts was a major obstacle to overcome, but it didn't even approach what followed. Eight months of chemo treatments took a toll on my outward appearance, leaving me pale, puffy, and hairless. "Face in the Mirror" provided the assurance that I could still look good despite any circumstances.

On another occasion, I was attending a survivor tea party where the founder and CEO of "Face in the Mirror" shared the story of the birth of this volunteer organization. Barbara MacLean had been visiting her sister, Charlotte McCracken, who was battling breast cancer. She offered to give her a facial to help lift her spirits and was surprised at the results. Barbara couldn't believe what a difference a simple make-over provided for her sister. Charlotte said, "Promise me you will do this for others." Barbara fulfilled that promise, creating a non-profit organization to provide free services and products for those suffering from the effects of cancer. I was a personal witness of the psychological strength this organization brought into my life during my cancer journey. "Face in the Mirror" has served countless cancer patients and I express thanks to Barbara MacLean and all those who selflessly volunteer, as well as to those who donate the products that remind us we are still women.

Another organization that aided my process in healing was "Casting for Recovery." I first learned about CFR from an email forwarded by my cancer center's counselor. One of the cancer survivors in our support group had attended a retreat and raved about her experience. I immediately went to Casting for Recovery's website to learn more. This nationwide organization was founded in 1996 in Manchester, Vermont, by a breast cancer reconstructive surgeon and a professional fly fisher. I learned that their mission was to promote healing by providing breast cancer patients with the tools necessary to live a full life despite their diagnosis. I couldn't imagine how fly fishing and breast cancer could be related, but I was curious enough to read on. I already knew that being outdoors was therapeutic, but I learned that the very act of casting a fishing rod was similar to the exercises surgeons recommend after surgery to promote soft tissue stretching.

The more I read, the more I was convinced I wanted to benefit from this experience which was being held in my area at the Whispering Pines Resort in Pinetop, Arizona. I learned that two retreats were held each year, one in October and one in May. My teaching job prohibited me from attending the May event, but my Fall Break fell right during the October dates. I eagerly submitted all the necessary paperwork and waited for a response.

Only fourteen participants are selected randomly from the pool of applicants. I was disappointed to learn that I was chosen as an alternate for the October retreat. I was sure this meant I wouldn't be able to go this year. I put the matter out of my mind, determined to apply again at a later date. Imagine my surprise when just two weeks before the event, I received a call from a representative informing me that an opening had occurred and I was the first alternate. I was asked if I would be interested in attending and I almost turned the opportunity down, having made different plans for my Fall break.

Hesitantly, I accepted, trying to quickly adjust the plans in my head. How grateful I am that I didn't turn down this amazing experience.

The volunteer directed me to the website where I found a list of items to bring and the schedule of events. I read some testimonials of past participants and my excitement grew. Since Pinetop is three hours from our home in Mesa, Randy planned to stay in the area after dropping me off at the resort and enjoy the beautiful outdoors as well. We both were adjusting nicely to this unexpected turn of events.

As the days approached my excitement increased and I eagerly gathered all I needed. I even managed to tie a fleece blanket printed with the pink breast cancer symbol for my roommate. I didn't know her yet, but I knew she would be special.

When Randy and I arrived at the main cabin in Pinetop on the first day of the retreat, we were greeted by a staff of friendly and energetic women. I was given a schedule of events for the next few days, a Casting for Recovery hat, and the opportunity to mingle with and meet the women who would soon become dear friends.

After spending some time at the welcoming reception, Randy and I decided to find my assigned cabin and drop off my luggage. I was hoping to meet my roommate who wasn't among those at the reception. I was pleased to find that my cabin, nestled among the beautiful pines of northern Arizona, was located close to the main cabin and hub of activity. I still had an issue with walking long distances so this would be perfect.

Randy carried my luggage up the wooden steps to the cabin's door, decorated with a large pink breast cancer ribbon. As I pushed to open the door, I discovered it was locked. I could hear voices inside, so I knocked until a man finally heard me and apologetically opened the door. It was my roommate's husband and he explained how his wife always felt safer with the door locked. This didn't surprise me as I had learned about the various degrees of anxieties that affect a cancer patient. I had a few of my own. Excited to meet my roommate, I walked in.

Mary was short in stature and very shy. Besides her husband, she was accompanied by a daughter who appeared to be about nine years old. After brief introductions, her husband and daughter left. Randy followed, anxious to check into his own place, and allow me to settle and begin my experience.

I tried to start a conversation with Mary, but she just showed me the empty room which was to be mine, and disappeared into her own room. After I unpacked a few things, I walked to the window. The view was breathtaking. Before me stood a forest of majestic pine trees, with a perfectly shaped tree so close to the cabin, the branches brushed my window. The ground was scattered with hundreds of pine cones and I made a mental note to gather some to take back to my students.

I opened the window and slowly inhaled the fragrant pine-scented air. A cool breeze rustled the pine boughs slightly, creating a calm, peaceful sound. Participating in this retreat and being in these surroundings was going to be just what I needed.

I checked the schedule of events and realized it was almost time to be back at the main lodge for an activity and dinner. Mary seemed busy in her room, but I knocked softly on the door and invited her to walk down with me. She seemed ready to get to know me so we visited a few minutes in the cabin, sharing a little bit about our cancer and where we were in the healing process. Before leaving for dinner, however, she pointed out a front cabin window that wouldn't close completely, keeping it from locking into place. I could tell that bothered her so I tried to fix it, but to no avail. I ended up propping a stick against it, assuring her that would help until we could report the problem. Luckily, she agreed, allowing us to proceed forward to the evening's events. Mary wanted to lock the front door, but I reminded her that neither of us had a key to get back in. I assured her all would be safe.

Later I found out there was a good reason we didn't have keys and our doors remained unlocked. Every time we returned to our cabins after a gathering, we discovered thoughtful little gifts on our pillows, delivered by some mysterious staff member. This tender act of kindness was just one example of what was in store for the fourteen breast cancer survivors chosen for this retreat.

Some of my readers may have the opportunity to attend a Casting for Recovery event and so I will purposely leave out the details of my memorable days in the pines. Each participant deserves to experience the element of surprise awaiting them at this well-orchestrated retreat.

We spent an amazing three days making new friends, sharing fears and concerns, learning to properly cast a fly-fishing rod, and applying our newly acquired knowledge at a nearby lake with a volunteer expert fisherman. We all received physical and emotional healing in a setting of peace and beauty with the help of the staff and guest speakers.

In addition to all I learned, I grew to love Mary. She eventually trusted me enough to open her heart and we shared some incredible moments of self-discovery together. On the last day, I placed the blanket I made on her pillow with a note of love and appreciation for the time we shared. I let her know it was meant to comfort her in the months ahead and be a reminder of our friendship. We parted as dear friends who shared things that most others in our lives don't understand.

Twice a year, Patricia from the hospital breast cancer support group organizes a function entitled "Day of Art." It was always in November and April, making it impossible for me to attend due to my teaching responsibilities. The first year after my retirement in 2014, I signed up to participate. We could bring someone along who assisted us on our cancer journey and I chose my daughter Kristy, who not only was a great support but a talented artist.

I thought a lot about what I would paint that would adequately describe my cancer experience. Maybe a lantern or candle radiating light, a rainbow of hope, or perhaps a butterfly of freedom. I remembered my stay in the hospital after surgery to remove cancer, and the labored walk down the hall lined with pictures. Those paintings were from the Day of Art, all created by cancer patients. Now it was my turn to inspire and uplift and I desperately wanted my painting to pay suitable homage to my cancer journey.

Prior to my turn at the November Day of Art, I had attended a conference in which Dieter F. Uchtdorf, a leader in my Church, gave a talk that touched me deeply. He spoke of our tendency to put up umbrellas of fear and doubt which block the many blessings that our Heavenly Father is constantly raining upon us. We need to have the faith to close our umbrellas and accept these blessings. This message rang true as I thought of my umbrella of fear and doubt that I held tightly to protect me from the effects of my cancer journey. I decided to paint myself in a rainstorm with my arms outstretched, inviting the downpour, with my umbrella tossed aside.

Kristy and I arrived at our Day of Art to find several friends from previous encounters, a colorful array of acrylic paints, brushes and spatulas, and a large canvas for each participant. The day flew by as I attempted to paint on canvas the picture in my head. Kristy assisted me with some technical details, but the painting was mine and the end result was a true expression of my cancer experience as seen with my heart. I penned the following words to go with my creation.

> *We all experience storms in our lives. Our immediate reaction is to quickly get out our umbrellas to shield us from the onslaught of rain. That is what I naturally did when I was diagnosed with stage-three breast cancer. My umbrella of fear, disbelief, and confusion protected me from getting soaked all at once, but it also shielded me from the blessings in disguise that storms can bring. With time, I learned to trust enough to set my umbrella aside and allow all the blessings and important lessons soak in that I needed to learn. Lessons of self-discovery, trusting in God, gratitude for each new day, and a deeper love and appreciation for my family, are a few of the important things I gained from my cancer experience. Probably the most difficult lesson was setting aside the fear of cancer returning and trusting that if it does, it will be alright. In the beginning, we need our umbrellas because the storms of cancer hit unexpectedly, but the sooner we muster up the courage to throw aside our protective coverings, the sooner we can participate in all the good things that the storms of life bring.*

For one year, my painting hung on a wall in the hospital, just like the ones I saw at the beginning of my cancer journey. I was now able to inspire and lift someone whose journey had just begun. Having the opportunity to contribute my own creation completed the circle.

I owe much to the many volunteers and organizations that have smiled upon me and have given me courage and the tools necessary to continue my cancer journey with grace. I owe much to the friends that have held my hand and given me a push when necessary. All of them have impacted my heart and have been instruments in my quest to overcome the adversities I have faced since the day I first learned I had cancer. To you I pay deep respect and gratitude.

*August 24, 2015*

*Dear Journal,*

*Fear is an interesting opponent. You think you've defeated it only to find it has been dormant, cleverly waiting for a reason to resurface. I feel somewhat justified in my inability to eliminate the fear of cancer returning. Having hormone receptor positive breast cancer means it can find another place in my body to reside, without prior notice or giving a forwarding address. Cancer is fickle and I can't control it, but I can manage fear and its influence on my thoughts and actions.*

*My dilemma is that I've been trying to figure out how to accomplish this for the last six years.*

14

# THE FEAR SYNDROME

It has been six years since I sat in a waiting room draped with a pink paper gown, anticipating the worst, hoping for the best. Now I find myself draped similarly, but the gown is white and I am perched on the end of an exam table at my routine six-month visit with Dr. Polowy. The scene has become a familiar one for me. Dr. Polowy strolls in with his big grin and friendly greeting. I am asked a series of questions and as I answer them, he is gently going through his routine of making sure there are no changes in the surgical area. It is my turn to go over the questions that have formulated in my mind over the last six months, and he listens carefully, never in a hurry, responding patiently. As he leaves, he turns and asks, "How is your book coming?" "Almost done," I answer. "Except for the ending. I'm having trouble with the ending."

That was an understatement. I was struggling with more than one ending, the most significant, putting an end to fear. As soon as I thought I was making progress, a new concern would creep into my life, and the fear of cancer returning swept over me like a thick cloud of dust, blinding my ability to think logically.

Before my cancer diagnosis, I completely trusted my body. I had no reason not to. It had always been my ally, my best friend, allowing me to fulfill the longings of my energetic spirit. As long as I treated it like a good buddy, giving it proper nutrition and resting between my long lists of projects, it would allow me to pursue whatever I wanted. I had enjoyed optimum health for the first 58 years of my life. I had given life to six healthy babies using natural childbirth techniques, and I always recovered quickly with the energy needed to take care of a large family. When I first noticed the distortion of my left nipple, I didn't even consider it to be a problem. I ignored the warning signs, never believing my body would ever let me down.

For most people diagnosed with cancer it comes as a complete surprise. The unsuspecting victim is living a normal, happy life, oblivious to the silent storm brewing within. A trip to the doctor for a minor complaint suddenly results in a verdict of cancer. BAM. Your life's course has suddenly changed. My reaction to this was to be proactive. Cancer would never have the chance to creep into my life again.

Unfortunately, this approach results in a great deal of unnecessary worry about any unusual ache, no matter how small and insignificant. I became overly concerned about my body, mentioning every minor symptom I experienced during my visits with Dr. Polowy. I don't know how he put up with my constant worry, but I have to credit him for his patience and ability to put my concerns to rest. When he thought my complaint was significant, he ordered scans or imaging. Otherwise he would assure me that what I was experiencing was normal, calming my fears without being judgmental. I always felt guilty for being so anxious and apprehensive. As much as I tried, I couldn't shake the worry of cancer reappearing at the most inconvenient moment. Fear had me in a tight grip.

It was the same every time. I would approach the date of my routine check-up with Dr. Polowy, hopeful that I could proclaim, "no questions, no worries." However, as the day of the appointment drew closer, a new symptom would manifest itself that I felt worthy of consideration. I'd decide we'd better check to be absolutely sure that my latest ailment was not an indication of cancer returning to spin my world out of control.

One time it was a persistent cough, another was throbbing in my ribs. This time it was pain in my back. I had started experiencing a sharp, stabbing ache down my spine, just below my shoulder blades. It would worsen as the day went on, sometimes making it difficult to fall asleep. I tried several methods of handling this new development such as exercising and being more conscious of proper posture. The backaches continued, worsening with time. I weighed the pros and cons of mentioning it at my next visit with Dr. Polowy. I had read that if cancer metastasizes to the bone, it will most often be manifested by traces of calcium found in the blood. If my blood results were normal, I decided not to mention my back pain but save my concerns for my Primary Care Provider. I found that as in past cases, my anxiety was concentrated more on apprehension of cancer returning than on the actual need to treat the problem. Most of all, I didn't want to approach Dr. Polowy with yet another concern, and I didn't want to schedule more imaging. I was trying desperately to appear confident that my health had finally returned to the status of "Excellent". Or at least "Very Good".

My resolve was short-lived, however. Before seeing Dr. Polowy, his nurse practitioner entered the exam room and asked me a barrage of questions, one being if I was experiencing any bone pain. Without thinking, I mentioned the pain in my back, which she noted. Realizing what I had said, I quickly asked if my blood work was normal. She remarked that it was great, and I was instantly sorry that I mentioned the back pain. She excused herself, leaving me alone in the room to wait for Dr. Polowy. I thought the matter was over so I was surprised that it was the first topic of discussion when my oncologist entered the exam room.

"So I hear you have been experiencing some pain in your back. Tell me about it."

"Well, it seems to be concentrated in the middle of my back between my shoulder blades and is unlike muscle pain that I sometimes feel in my lower back. I'm not sure how to tell the difference between bone and muscle pain, but this pain seems to be directly in my spine."

After feeling down my back and having me guide him to where it was most uncomfortable, he remarked, "Well I would feel better if we schedule a full body bone scan. The chances of cancer metastasizing to the spine are slim, but I want to check it out."

My heart sank upon hearing those words. Another scan, another waiting for results, another worry, and I didn't like the words, "full body". Why not just the spine? Since Dr. Polowy was concerned, I became even more concerned and lost my head as I began to spout off every little health issue that might be related to my back pain over the last six months. Dr. Polowy had to be a little surprised at my list of ailments and responded with, "I want to see you again in three months."

This was not what I wanted to hear. After striving to trust my body again, I was back at square one, revealing my insecurities. I went in hoping that my next appointment would move from six months to one year, not from six months to three months, and the last thing I wanted was another imaging appointment. I left the office wondering how long it was going to take to overcome my fear of finding more cancer.

As I drove home, I decided that if I did follow through and make an appointment for a bone scan, I wouldn't mention it to anyone, especially Randy. I was done dragging him through the days of worry, waiting for results. If it was possible for anyone to worry more than me, it was him. Since this was most likely just a check to be sure, there was no need to alarm him or anyone else.

If I had to call and make the appointment for my bone scan, it probably would not have happened. As it was, the imaging center called me and the appointment was set for the following Monday morning. I reasoned that I could still cancel at any time.

When I received instructions for my appointment, I was surprised to hear that I would be required to come in the morning and receive an injection before returning to have the scan three hours later. This was different than my last bone scan five years earlier. I decided to look up bone scans on the internet to learn about these changes, as well as more information about back and bone pain. Rule number one: Do not go on the internet to research health issues.

Wikipedia was very informative with their explanation of what I could expect with my scheduled scan. The radioactive material they would be injecting would indicate areas that were affected by cancer. It included a skeletal picture of a patient's scan that showed multiple bone metastases resulting from prostate cancer. The cancerous areas were visibly darker.

In addition, I began reading about what symptoms were associated with bone pain, especially in the spine. I could relate with many of them, although I was reminded that the pain I was experiencing could mean several different problems, not related to cancer. Still, I was becoming more convinced that I should go ahead with the scheduled appointment, just to make sure.

I arrived at the imaging center early Monday morning to receive my injection as scheduled. The technician and I immediately connected, having discovered we went to the same high school years ago. I was glad to hear she would be there when I returned three hours later to perform the scan. I busied myself with housework to help the time go by quickly, returning at noon, confident that this was just a matter of caution and all would be fine.

The bone scan itself was brief, lasting no more than fifteen minutes. I was amazed at how different it was from my last experience five years ago. The technician remained in the room and when I stood up from the narrow table, I could see the images of my skeleton on four separate computer screens.

I was distressed to see that the last screen showed my entire spine darkened like the picture I saw on the internet. There was also a dark spot on my skull, as well as my pelvis. I was expecting the pelvis to be dark as I had read that the radioactive material leaves the body through the kidneys and bladder in urine, but was shocked to see the spine and skull appearing black. I immediately concluded from this observation that indeed cancer had spread to my spine and perhaps my brain as well. Rule number two: Never try to interpret the results of your imaging. This takes intensive training.

After my scan, the technician seemed different. Her previous friendly demeanor was replaced by a sober countenance and she attempted to distract me from staring at the computer screens by commenting on how much she liked my purse. Rule number three: Don't try to read the technician.

I drove home in shock. From what I could see, my entire spine had been affected by cancer, as well as my brain. No wonder the buzzing in my ears had intensified in the last six months. The next three days were filled with grief and fear of what the future would bring as I waited for the results to be confirmed. I was convinced that my breast cancer had metastasized, and since I hadn't told anyone of the bone scan, I worried alone. I thought of how I would break the news to Randy and my family. I wondered if I would be required to endure more chemotherapy. How many more years would I live? I must admit, I was getting a bit dramatic.

After the third fretful day of waiting passed and I hadn't heard from Dr. Polowy or his nurse, I decided to call and see if the office had received the results. I was encouraged by the fact that I didn't hear immediately, which might mean that things weren't as bad as I thought. I had to leave a message at the nurse's desk which meant I now had to wait for a call back. Waiting for this call was painful.

I decided to go about my day as planned, but I was jittery and restless. In about an hour I was scheduled to pick up my granddaughter for her birthday sleepover and shopping trip. How I wanted to hear back before this activity began. I had suffered three days of worry and was understandably anxious to hear from my doctor.

I jumped when the phone finally rang. I was in a store so I quickly walked outside before answering. My heart was racing with anticipation at what I was about to hear. I was trying hard to be brave and take the expected news with grace.

"Hi, is this Claudia?"

"Yes, it is."

"This is Jan from Dr. Polowy's office. I'm returning your call concerning the results of your bone scan." As she paused to take a breath, my heart raced, imagining how this was going to sound. As she continued, I strained to make sure I was hearing her correctly. "I'm happy to tell you that there was no bone cancer found, just some degenerative disks in the spine that are a result of aging. Do you have any questions?"

"No. Thank you so much for the good news!" Relief swept over me as I realized how wrong I had been about my scan. I felt a little ridiculous for the unnecessary suffering I went through, thinking I could interpret the results of a bone scan by looking at a picture on Wikipedia. My gratitude upon hearing I was still cancer free was mixed with disgust at my inability to move forward, free of the fear that was consuming my life. I had gone through a week of unnecessary anxiety and I was losing patience with the cancer ghost that had won another victory, laughing all the way.

Why was I having such a difficult time with this? I envied my friend Shawna, another breast cancer survivor, who would assure me, "We are done with cancer, Claudia. When we die, it won't be from cancer." How could she be so sure? What was her secret? I wanted desperately to have that kind of assurance, that kind of faith.

After much self-evaluation, I identified some legitimate causes that helped justify my fear. Number one on my list—my favorite aunt died from breast cancer. I remember Aunt

Millie, who was married to my mom's brother, being diagnosed when I was still a young mother. She endured rounds of chemo, lost her hair, and was declared cancer free after her treatments were completed. We were all relieved that she was healed. She faithfully took Tamoxifen for the full five years, only to have the cancer metastasize to her lungs. She was five years out and it came back. It continued to spread and she passed away after a painful battle.

In comparison, I didn't take the recommended hormone therapy for more than twelve months. With my percentage of survival lowered, was I setting myself up for a similar outcome?

I made a lot of friends during my cancer journey, meeting them at support meetings and during my months of chemotherapy. When I would see one of them return to treatments due to reoccurrence, I would wonder, why them? We had a similar cancer, similar treatment. Why does cancer return for some and not others? I don't think the doctors even know the answer to that question.

I have a large painted wooden sign in my home that says one word: "BELIEVE". I purchased it to hang during the Christmas holidays, but has remained hanging year-round for the last three years, encouraging me to do just that. What does it take to truly believe that my health has been restored, that I am a survivor, and that I can move forward with confidence in the future? How do I clear my mind of negative, crippling thoughts? Is there any hope for such a doubter?

Something needed to change or I would be spending the rest of my life anticipating the eventual invasion of that one escapee that may be lurking in my body, or maybe just in my mind.

It's hard to let go of the memory of the day I learned I had cancer. I felt violated, betrayed, and confused. My desperate fear of a repeat performance was clouding my judgment and ability to live without always looking over my shoulder for that cancer demon.

Since being declared cancer free, I recognized an undesirable pattern of fear that remained to haunt me. I asked myself over and over, *How do I break the pattern and develop sufficient faith to get me through the next scare?*

It's easy to have faith when all is going smoothly. The test of faith comes when once again I am face to face with another health issue that warrants consideration. My heart understands and believes that God is in charge, and I know He loves me and wants me to be happy. If I could get my mind and heart to be in harmony with that knowledge, maybe I could finally break the tightening vise of fear.

*January 19, 2016*

*What is going on? Without warning, I am lying in a hospital bed with an NG tube running down my nose and into my stomach. Imaging has shown enlarged lymph nodes in my abdomen. Dr. Polowy has been summoned and tests are being ordered.*

*I am a seven-year survivor so it certainly couldn't be cancer.*

*Or could it?*

15

# MORE THAN JUST SURVIVING

Four months had passed since my last scare of cancer returning. I was feeling great, sleeping better, and noticing a surge of vigor and purpose in life. My desire to move forward with hope and eliminate the crippling fear of the last six years motivated me to have positive thoughts and faith in my future. I felt like I was making progress but wondered if it was because I was feeling physically strong. We think we know ourselves, but in times of trial, we find out the truth. What would happen if another health issue presented itself? Was I really conquering fear, or would it raise its ugly head when a new challenge appeared? Even though my paradigm shift was untested, I was hopeful and optimistic, and beginning to feel more like the person I was before the cancer took control.

My story took a new twist as the world finished celebrating Christmas and the 2016 New Year festivities had settled into another boring, drab January. Randy and I decided to spice things up by taking a trip to Sedona, Arizona, just a few hours from our home in Mesa. I was feeling on top of the world, excited for all the things I had to look forward to in the upcoming year; a family reunion in March and our son's graduation from medical school in May. I was rejoicing in excellent health and the increased energy I was feeling. During our drive to the resort we had reserved, Randy and I made

New Year resolutions and talked about improvements we wished to make individually and together.

It was cold in Sedona, at least to an Arizona girl, but seeing the white snow on the red rocks was breathtaking. Soft daylight still prevailed when we entered the city and as we drove by different shops and restaurants, we verbally made plans for the week. I was excited for a relaxing change of scenery and planned to do some writing in the pines by the creek that ran past our dwelling.

After making a simple dinner of roasted chicken, butternut squash, and green salad the second evening of our stay, our blissful vacation quickly went sour. I barely got up from eating when I was hit with intense pain in my abdomen. I didn't say a word to Randy, hoping the pain would soon fade. What could this be? I already had my appendix out, yet the pain resembled appendicitis and spread across my lower abdomen. Doubled over and clutching my stomach, I went to the bedroom and laid down in a fetal position. I got up once to use the bathroom, but even that didn't help. A feeling of panic swept over me as I realized that something was terribly wrong.

In the meantime, Randy had finished eating and was putting away the leftover food. I called for him to come into the bedroom. He walked in, completely oblivious of my plight. You can imagine his shock when I groaned, "You need to take me to the Emergency Room."

I don't think I've ever said those words in my lifetime. I might have said, "Do you think we should go to the Emergency Room?" but never had I boldly declared the need to make such a trip without wondering if it was the right thing to do.

After trying to explain the intense pain, which was not going away, Randy sprang into action. Grabbing his iPhone, he asked Siri, "Where is the nearest hospital?" Despite my pain, I was amused watching the interchange between Randy and technology. Maybe it was his frantic tone of voice, or Siri's attitude, but she kept directing him to a non-related website, frustrating him beyond words. Between his futile attempts to locate a hospital, I tried to get his attention to let him know I knew the location of an Emergency Room in Sedona.

Repeating myself for the third time, he finally looked at me in disbelief. "How do you know where an Emergency Room is? I've never seen one all the times we've been here."

It just so happened that on our Sunday afternoon drive, I had spotted one on the right side of the road. I remembered making a mental note of it, never expecting the need for its services. I simply told Randy to take the same road we had driven earlier that day. Relieved that he didn't have to depend on his phone for directions, we grabbed jackets and my purse and headed out the door.

The drive took around fifteen minutes and in between praying for help to withstand the constant pain, I tried to logically determine what could be happening. Was I passing a kidney stone? I heard that was very much like childbirth. Having birthed six children, I was well acquainted with intense pain. Perhaps it was a gall bladder attack, or a blockage in my bowels. I will never forget my appendicitis attack twenty years ago. I was required to endure the pain for hours while the doctor tried to determine the cause. I wasn't given pain medication so as not to "mask the symptoms". I never could figure out the logic in that approach. I didn't think I could tolerate my current pain much longer and was horrified at the possibility of walking into a busy Emergency Room, going through the admittance process, and trying to endure an agonizing wait.

The Emergency Room soon came into view, right where I had seen it earlier that afternoon. Randy found a close parking spot and helped me into the building. Being astonished and relieved to see an empty waiting room, I struggled to walk to the admittance window. After a brief explanation of why I was there, the receptionist asked to see my driver's license and insurance card. It was all I could do to retrieve them from my wallet and toss them in her direction. I was taken to a room right away.

A nurse began an IV and I was immediately given pain medication. My intense pain apparently was obvious because they didn't bother to ask me to rate it on a scale of 1-10. After taking blood samples, they inquired about my pain, which had dulled but was not gone, so they offered something stronger. I agreed, and within minutes, I was finally able to relax.

I was informed that I would need a CT scan and blood work to help determine what was going on and was asked if I could give them a urine sample. By this point, it was easy to be compliant with their requests, having my initial pain relieved.

Gratitude overwhelmed me at the good fortune in having been served so quickly. As we waited for the results of the blood work and scan, we visited with the nurse and found that Sedona didn't have a hospital. This was only an Emergency Room and if I needed to be admitted I would be required to go by ambulance to the nearest hospital in Cottonwood. I was hoping that wouldn't be necessary.

Following a lengthy wait, a doctor walked in to visit with us about his findings. My blood work was absolutely normal and the only thing the CT scan showed were enlarged lymph nodes. There was no indication of a kidney stone, gall bladder problems, or bowel blockage. How strange. Hearing this brought a sense of relief, but also a sense of wonderment. What could be causing such acute pain? I'm not sure which is worse, knowing or not knowing what is wrong. At least when the problem is identified, a plan for correction can be made.

The doctor explained what I was experiencing could possibly be a viral infection that mimicked appendicitis. That seemed like a logical explanation. Since there was nothing more he could do, he released me with instructions to return if the pain continued. To help me through the night, I was given pain and nausea medication in pill form.

Returning to our resort, we got ready for bed. I took one of the pills provided by the doctor as the pain was returning with intensity. I tried to sleep, but the medication wasn't helping. I was told I could take up to two pain pills every four hours so after thirty minutes, I took another. Finding it still impossible to sleep, I tried to find a comfortable position and endure the long night ahead. After four hours, I took two more pills and was finally able to doze for about two hours. I awoke early, exhausted and still struggling with the pain. My restlessness aroused Randy and he asked, "How are you doing?"

"I've been up all night and I only have two pain pills left. Should we go back to the Emergency Room?"

"I think we need to pack up and get you down to Mesa. I'd rather you be at a familiar hospital if you have to be admitted."

It was 6:00 a.m. and by 7:00 a.m., Randy had packed all our belongings, the food we had brought, left the keys on the table, and we were on our way. Right before leaving, I took the last of the pain pills to get me through the two-hour drive.

I don't remember much about the trip back to Mesa. We visited very little and I would often pull my knees up to my chest, providing some comfort. I was amazed at the rapid change of events and was mystified as to the cause. One thing was for certain. Something was not right. Despite what last night's tests didn't show, there was something terribly wrong inside my abdomen. The regret I felt for our spoiled vacation was minimal compared to the fear I sensed about the unknown ahead.

When we arrived in Mesa, Randy decided to drive straight to the Emergency Room. Again, I was able to skip the wait and was admitted and given pain medication through an IV. It was like a rerun of the night before as the technicians obtained blood samples and I was whisked away for another CT scan.

While waiting to hear from a doctor concerning the test results, Randy received a text from our daughter Julie.

"Can you guys say a little prayer for Shiloh? We went to the park today to ride scooters and he fell and broke his wrist pretty badly. The bone apparently broke and then lifted up over the other bone. They sent us to Cardon Children's Hospital. Shiloh has been super brave! The pediatrician said it's a pretty painful break. So much for enjoying the nice weather!"

Shiloh was our five-year-old grandson and I cringed when I heard he broke his wrist riding the scooter we bought him for Christmas. To make this even more interesting, Cardon Children's Hospital was part of Banner Desert Hospital where I was being treated. My daughter and grandson were just down the hall. I could hardly wait to make my presence known, which would be a shock as our family expected us to be in Sedona having a wonderful vacation. What are the odds that we would be at the same hospital at the same time?

Randy sent Julie a quick text announcing our presence and asking for their room number. Julie responded, completely astonished with the news of my illness and our thwarted vacation. Randy left to visit them, excited to check on our grandson and bring Julie up to date.

After a wait of several hours, the doctor came in to report the same results found in Sedona. I was thankful to hear nothing serious was discovered, but I was baffled as to why I was experiencing so much pain. Could enlarged lymph nodes cause the degree of discomfort I was experiencing? The doctor said he would like to keep me overnight to manage the pain, and as soon as a bed was available, I would be moved to the observation ward. Due to my history and discovering a change in the lymph nodes, he had contacted Dr. Polowy. By now I was accustomed to the check, recheck, and double check given to a patient who has ever had cancer.

It was evening by the time I was taken to my room and I hadn't eaten for twenty-four hours. I ordered dinner, most of which Randy ate. I thought I was hungry, but the little bit I got down didn't settle well. Besides, right after dinner was brought, Julie and Shiloh entered for hugs and a quick visit. I thought it was pretty special to have shared an emergency room experience together, and Shiloh couldn't stop grinning. After everyone left, I tried to find a comfortable position on the hospital bed. I love to play with the controls that can raise and lower the feet and head until it feels just right. Since I had little sleep the night before and was administered pain medication through my IV, I slept comfortably.

Morning brought one of the friendliest nurses I've ever had, more blood work, breakfast, and a visit from Dr. Polowy. It was comforting to know he was aware of what was going on, and he reassured me of the unlikelihood of cancer. As he sat by the bed and visited about my symptoms, he didn't seem overly concerned, but shared that he had ordered blood work to check for tumor markers. I knew it was just a matter of procedure and didn't worry.

Later that morning, the hospitalist came in to check on my progress and saw no reason to keep me in the hospital. I was in total agreement and called Randy with the good news. After the nurse removed my IV, I dressed and waited on the bed for Randy to arrive. As I sat there, I noticed the pain in my abdomen gradually returning. This concerned me. What was I supposed to do if the abdominal pain became severe? I asked the nurse if the doctor had left a prescription for pain medicine. Finding he hadn't and explaining how I was feeling, she agreed to locate him and ask. I was relieved that by the time Randy arrived, the nurse had contacted the doctor and I was granted my request.

Arriving home, I ate a simple lunch and rested on our recliner sofa. Randy made a run to the store to purchase the only things I felt like eating—chicken noodle soup and saltine crackers. Kristy, now living in Arizona, came over with my three-year-old grandson, Gage, who helped distract me from the mounting pain. I laughed at Gage who, noticing that all my Christmas decorations were still up, declared, "Grandma, it isn't Christmas anymore!" I had decided to pack away Christmas after returning from our vacation in Sedona, a decision I later regretted. It would be quite some time before I could put away my holiday decorations.

As evening approached, I found it necessary to take some of the pain medication the doctor had prescribed upon leaving the hospital. Since it had to be taken with food, I tried to eat a few crackers, but even they didn't settle well. As the evening wore on, the pain increased to its original intensity, but this time I experienced nausea. We discussed returning to the Emergency Room, but first decided to call our son, a fourth-year medical student, for advice. While Randy talked to him on the phone, I ran to the bathroom and threw up several times. This reduced the pain in my abdomen and I elected to try and make it through the night. The last thing I wanted was to return to the Emergency Room, and clung to any sliver of improvement to avoid another trip. Taking my last nausea pill, I tried to get some sleep.

The night went better than I expected and when I awoke I felt I could tolerate some food. I ate a whole slice of bread and drank some Gatorade. Grateful that I had escaped another trip to the hospital, I rested on the couch, hopeful that I was on the mend.

Sharing my relief, Randy put on a movie to help pass the morning. As we watched, I noticed the pain was once again returning. Slowly at first, allowing room for hope, but soon escalating to the point of intolerable pain. I didn't have to say anything, as one look told Randy the drama was not over.

Instinctively, I knew something was wrong with my body, despite the negative test results. Since the discharge papers said to call my primary care physician in the event of further symptoms, I complied, only to be told I needed to go to the Emergency Room. As I threw on a few clothes, nausea hit, sending me to the bathroom. Once I again I vomited the contents of my stomach.

I do not like the ER. Only under dire circumstances would I face that kind of punishment, three times in three days. What else could I do? I was not able to withstand the pain, and I could think of no other alternative.

Checking in, it was obvious to the front desk that I had been a frequent visitor. Glancing up from the computer, the receptionist looked skeptical as she took my insurance card. I was not received with the same courtesy or compassion as before. As the technician walked me to a vacant cubicle she handed me a cup.

"We need a urine sample."

"I can't go right now. I haven't been able to keep anything down for the last twenty-four hours."

"Your kidneys are always producing urine. We need a sample now", she curtly replied.

Fortunately, the restroom was occupied, so I was allowed to change into a gown and lie on a bed. After taking my vitals, the technician looked at me and snapped, "Your temperature is normal." Throughout this whole adventure, I never had a fever, which stumped the doctors, especially since the symptoms pointed toward an infection. My white blood count was also normal, not indicative of an infection. Tossing the thermometer cover into the garbage, my ever so friendly technician reminded me of the urine sample as he walked out of the room.

By the time the restroom was empty, I was able to grant them a small amount of urine. Having had two CT scans on my previous visits, the doctor ordered an X-Ray. This time, the results came back quickly as they discovered a blockage in my bowel. With a cause determined, the staff became more tolerant of my presence. Although I didn't like the diagnosis, I was relieved that there was finally some explanation for my pain.

Hearing them assign a surgeon to my case, I spoke up and requested Dr. Deyden, someone I knew and trusted. I wasn't sure if they would comply, but it didn't hurt to voice my desire and build the team that would be making the decisions. I was informed that an NG tube would be placed. I had no idea what that was, but would soon find out. A nurse came in and asked if I would mind having a student, with her guidance, place the NG tube. Knowing my own son in medical school would gain experience this way once he was a resident, I innocently agreed.

After explaining the procedure, the nurse gave a few last-minute instructions to the student. I was beginning to see that this was not going to be pleasant. A long, narrow tube would be inserted through my nose, down my throat and esophagus, and into my stomach. I could help the process by swallowing water through a straw while the student quickly shoved the tube down. After being asked which nostril I would like to use, (as if it mattered) and having been given something to numb the inside of my nose, they began. The nurse coached the student with encouraging remarks like, "Go faster! You still have a ways to go," while I frantically swallowed. Finally, the tube was in place. My throat ached with a foreign object present and I was disappointed to find they weren't going to remove it anytime soon. This also meant I wouldn't be allowed to eat or drink, and it hurt to talk. I tried not to focus on the dark green contents of my stomach, now flowing through the tube which was attached to a machine, constantly pumping.

I was transported to a room on the third floor by late afternoon. How ironic that in three days the view out my window transformed from the beautiful red rocks of Sedona to construction scaffolding populated by a flock of pigeons. It was my fortune to be in the section of the hospital that was being renovated. I can imagine I was also paying more per day for my room than the lovely resort we had to abandon, and unlike Sedona, my mobility was severely limited.

Before I could use the restroom, a nurse would have to be summoned to detach the NG tube from the pump and seal it closed. Maneuvering my IV pole in the small room wasn't easy, especially since I needed my free arm to hold together the back of my hospital gown which loved to gape open. The crowning event of the day was not being able to order dinner. The last complete meal I had was three evenings ago and since my pain was under control, I was hungry. Maybe that was a good sign.

On the second day in my new surroundings, I called the nurse to unhook my NG tube from the pumping machine so I could use the bathroom. A nurse's aide came and decided she could handle it since the nurses were busy. Grabbing my IV pole, I made my way around the bed, past the window, and into the small bathroom. This was a tricky process, especially since the IV pole wouldn't fit in the bathroom, unless I didn't close the door. Desiring some privacy, I elected to leave the pole outside, slipping the long tubing under the door and being careful not to move too abruptly and yank out my IV needle.

I decided to brush my teeth, bending over to find my toothbrush in the bag Randy had brought. How nice that my bad was already packed from our vacation, with more than I could possibly need for my hospital stay.

As I straightened, I felt a gooey liquid on my arm. It didn't take long to realize that my NG tube was leaking, and the brownish green gunk was dripping down my arm and spotting my hospital gown. I was wearing the contents of my stomach.

Making my way out of the tight bathroom, I pushed the nurses' call button. When the voice answered, I wasn't sure how I was going to phrase my dilemma. Trying not to sound panicked I muttered, "My NG tube is leaking. I'll need another gown and help cleaning this up." I noticed there were also drops on the floor.

After wiping the sticky slime off my arm with a paper towel, I gathered my gown in my left arm, pulling it up around my waist to catch further leaks. Using my right arm, I pushed the IV pole around to the foot of the bed which was adjacent to the large window in my room. My goal was to meet the nurse so she could properly seal the NG tube before clean up began. Waiting in this precarious position I glanced up to see not more than six feet away, two construction workers outside my window. Not having a free hand to close my blinds, I shrank back into the bathroom to await help.

Clean up was awkward due to difficulty in maneuvering a tube coming out of my nose along with an IV attached to my arm. The nurse helped me change the gown, and I was finally back in my bed, worn out from the experience. I didn't even get to brush my teeth.

During the next three days, I had the pleasure of two X-Ray sessions, one lasting nearly three hours. A considerable amount of liquid was forced down my NG tube into my stomach and multiple X-Rays were taken every fifteen to thirty minutes to watch the progress through my intestines. Dr. Polowy ordered an MRI, and Dr. Deyden an ultrasound of every organ in my abdomen. My two favorite, highly capable doctors were working together once again in my behalf. They each had different ideas about what imaging might lead to a diagnosis. As a result, I was a recipient of every scan the hospital offered, some more than once. The one scan that was left out was a PET scan which was not available at the hospital. Dr. Polowy assured me that he still wanted one after I was discharged. I could fill a photo album with pictures of my insides.

Several things were learned from these scans. The X-ray marathon indicated that the blockage self-corrected, and the ultrasound didn't find anything amiss with the organs in my abdomen. The MRI showed an area of my small intestine that was enlarged, but that was the only unusual finding. It seemed obvious to me that I was cured and it was time to be discharged. Unfortunately, the symptoms were still present with the addition of my abdomen being exceedingly bloated. Dr. Deyden took one look at me and declared, "You are not going home." He added to my dismay when he said with that characteristic twinkle in his eye, "You are a mystery."

Since the X-rays proved matter was coursing properly through my intestines, Dr. Deyden ordered the removal of the NG tube. Despite the discomfort in pulling the long apparatus back up through my throat and nose, I was delighted to be free of it. I was connected to one less device and it made showering less complicated.

By Saturday morning, Dr. Deyden decided he would perform laparoscopic surgery to clear away the scar tissue from my appendectomy that may have caused the blockage. He seemed indecisive, so scheduled the procedure for Monday, hoping everything would improve over the weekend and surgery wouldn't be needed. He told me to eat a normal diet as he wanted to see how my bowels would react. I was grateful I could eat, but the discomfort in my abdomen prevented me from enjoying food and I consumed very little.

On Sunday evening, I received a call from Dr. Deyden. He seemed disturbed that my situation hadn't changed for the better and decided to do one more CT scan in the morning. If everything looked normal, surgery would be cancelled and I could be discharged. I wasn't happy to have another imaging scheduled and seriously considered refusing. What was the point? The last two CT scans revealed little in the search for a diagnosis. Why subject myself to more radiation? I had already been through so much and I was ready to go home. I asked Randy to take a walk with me to help clear my mind. As I pushed my IV pole and shuffled through the halls of the hospital, I decided on a plan. I needed to make one of two choices. I could agree to the additional CT scan and see if the results produced any new clues, or I could bypass it and ask to be discharged. Time would disclose if I was cured. The problem with that scenario was the fear of the pain returning and having to begin again at square one, which would be the Emergency Room. I decided to sleep on it and make my decision in the morning.

That night I had a dream. It was a simple dream, concise and to the point. I was sitting on the edge of my hospital bed and a nurse walked in and handed me a piece of paper. On it were written the words, "It's a good thing we did the CT scan. Give me a call." The note was from Dr. Deyden.

The next morning, I was awakened early by my nurse who flipped on the lights and informed me I had one hour to drink a half gallon of thick liquid. I reminded her I wasn't to have anything to eat or drink after midnight in the event surgery would be required. She smiled and said this didn't count. It was a necessary preparation for my CT scan. It was then I remembered the dream, and I complied with a request that would normally annoy me. The first glassful was easy to get down as I was terribly thirsty. I had forty-five minutes to drink the final three cups. Choking down the last bit of liquid in the remaining five minutes was a challenge. If I wasn't nauseated and sick to my stomach before drinking the solution, I certainly was now.

It wasn't long before someone from transport came to take me for the CT scan. They weren't wasting any time. Even though I drank a liquid contrast, I was still administered another contrast through my IV. Making sure I was comfortable, the imaging began, this time taking far longer than any CT scan I've experienced. Noticing the differences, I was hopeful that if there was something amiss, it would be discovered.

Returning to my room, I tried to rest and process the early morning events. I thought of questions I should ask Dr. Deyden upon my discharge today. I was optimistic that the results of this scan would rule out any problem and I could go home. All other imaging had produced no clues, and I didn't expect this one to be different than previous results despite my dream. I decided I would take a shower and freshen up before my trip home. The only problem was I didn't feel like making the effort, so I closed my eyes and dozed.

I'm not sure how much time passed between returning from the CT scan and Dr. Deyden bursting into my room. I know that I wasn't expecting to see him so soon. I can only remember some of what he reported as the information was completely different than what I expected and my mind was running behind, trying to catch up with my doctor's animated account.

The radiologist had shown Dr. Deyden the images from the CT scan and it was discovered that something was attacking the wall of my small intestine. Present were lymph nodes, and two spots that looked suspicious. While in my room, Dr. Deyden called Dr. Polowy to report his findings, and they both agreed surgery was necessary.

As soon as Dr. Deyden left my room, I was told transport was here to take me to prepare for surgery. I wanted to text Randy and let him know of their decision, but there wasn't time. Looking at the nurse, I asked if she could let my husband know where to find me when he arrived. I didn't even have time to take that shower I wanted.

In Pre-Op, I was given a clean hospital gown, socks for my feet, and the familiar covering for my head. Once clad in surgery attire, and settled in a small room, Randy walked in. I tried to relate all that Dr. Deyden had said, answering his questions the best I could. He seemed quiet and thoughtful, and I asked if he was okay. "Give me some time. I'm trying to wrap this new information around in my head."

The anesthesiologist entered my cubicle, spending quite some time asking me questions. He looked at the IV in my arm remarking, "That is not going to work." It was the fourth IV inserted since my admission to the hospital and was leaking. Looking at my veins he said he would take care of that problem when I was under anesthesia. I thanked him profusely, not wanting to go through another battle with needles. This last insertion took quite some time and was done by one of the most experienced nurses on my floor, and even at that, wasn't working well.

Unlike my other experiences preparing for surgery, the wait was minimal, and before I was mentally ready, I was kissing Randy good-by while being rolled down the hall. After being pushed through two double doors leading into my operating room, I took in all that I could. It was very cold but I knew that soon wouldn't matter. The room was void of color, except for bright silver, from the counters to the table I was placed on, to the huge round light fixture above.

The last thing I remember was my anesthesiologist saying, "I'm giving you some oxygen, free of smell or taste, but for which you will be charged by the hospital." I liked his humor.

Oblivious to the happenings of the next few hours, I slowly awoke from surgery. I first noticed my eyes felt moist and were covered with what felt like bandages so I didn't attempt to open them. My lips were extremely dry and I licked them before asking if I could have something for the pain that racked my body. I never like waking up from surgery. My five senses are in overdrive, informing me that my body has been through a grueling journey while my mind slept.

I don't remember the trip back to my room, or being placed in my hospital bed. When I was coherent, I asked the nurse if she could wipe my eyes, which she did remarking, "I thought you were crying." "No", I answered thanking her. "They must have put an ointment around my eyes." Opening my eyes and noticing Randy was in the room I asked, "How long was the surgery?" He reported, "You were in there for two hours. Dr. Deyden removed six inches of your small intestine and it has been sent to pathology." He seemed weary.

Satisfied that all went well, I drifted off again until the nurse entered to administer pain medicine through my IV. That was the first time I noticed that the IV needle was in my neck. Not realizing it was a central line, I figured they had given up on my right arm. It was a bit awkward as the tubing was taped down in several places and covered with gauze. Of course, this meant I wouldn't be able to take a shower or wash my hair which was already past the point of disgusting. Submitting to this new development, I decided it did have its good points. I could bend my arm easily, and they could draw blood from it, eliminating the middle of the night visits from the lab, trying to find a vein in my hand. My right hand was one big bruise from the frequent blood draws.

Later that afternoon, Dr. Deyden poked his head into my room. He shared a few points from the surgery, repeating the removal of six inches of intestine and reporting he personally had gone to pathology to make sure they didn't miss a spot he found on the underneath portion. He seemed tired, and assured me they would have the results by Wednesday. Exclaiming how much better I was feeling, he smiled briefly, remarking, "Well, Claudia, you are on pain medicine." He reminded me I was not to eat or drink anything, as even the smallest sip of water could cause another blockage since my bowels were swollen. Asking how long before I could resume eating he stated, "Not until you pass gas or have a bowel movement."

I had already been in the hospital six days which exceeded any previous visit. It appeared my time here was not coming to an end soon. Even though I wanted to be home, I knew my body was not ready. I was being nourished strictly through IV fluids and I wasn't able to stand without assistance. My mind marveled at my dependence on this place and I willed to get better as soon as possible. At that moment, the thought of a bowel movement or even passing gas seemed nothing less than painful. I would need to accomplish some healing first.

That evening, Dr. Polowy came by to visit. Luckily Randy was still with me so he could hear what he had to say. I didn't realize it then, but as I look back, he had come to prepare us for the possibility of cancer. Unlike Dr. Deyden who always stood when he came, Dr. Polowy sat next to my bed. With his characteristic compassion, he first inquired about how I was feeling. His presence brought calmness and trust, knowing I was getting the best care available. Without wasting time, he calmly began with the purpose of his visit.

"If this is cancer, it is one of two possibilities. It could be lymphoma which we can take care of in a matter of a few weeks. The treatment is simple. I just treated a ninety-year-old woman with lymphoma and she did very well. There is also a possibility that your breast cancer has metastasized to the small intestine, which is rare, but I have seen it before. If that is the case, it is treatable, but not curable." The "not curable" part was said softly, under his breath.

Randy asked, "How do we know if the section of intestine that was removed has enough safe margins?"

"That only matters if the cancer is a primary one which doesn't occur on the intestine. It will either be lymphoma from the affected lymph nodes, or it will be a cancer that was already present that has metastasized."

I remember at this point, Randy took my hand and held it for the rest of the conversation. I was silent as Dr. Polowy answered a few other questions from Randy. Suddenly realizing how late it was, I remarked, "What are you doing working so late? Do you ever rest, or eat, or sleep?" Amazed at how vigilant this doctor was at providing his patients with the quality care and consideration they needed, regardless of the hour, I thanked him for his time. I sensed this was not an easy visit for him. He shook Randy's hand, and patted my arm which spoke volumes in his capacity to genuinely care for those he served.

Randy was deeply affected by Dr. Polowy's visit, but I didn't realize how much until later. He seemed worn out and asked if it would be all right if he left to go home. I was ready to get some sleep myself, and told him I would be just fine. Giving me a kiss, he walked out.

I tried to fall asleep, but instead reflected on our conversation with Dr. Polowy. I was surprised at my lack of concern about the possibility of this experience leading to a diagnosis of cancer. In the past, I was in a panic at the thought of my cancer metastasizing, and had endured a number of imaging appointments to rule it out in the years following my chemotherapy. What was different about this time, when the possibility was more real than ever? I was filled with peace as I told myself, "If this is cancer, then it is the path I'm supposed to take. I will accept whatever is meant to be." For the first time, and *finally*, I submitted to God's will. Before, I had desperately tried, but this time the resolve came from deep within my heart. It was genuine. It was real. I fell into a peaceful sleep.

The day after surgery was pretty mundane. I was encouraged by the nurses to walk, and even though I was still on pain medication administered through my IV, getting out of bed was the last thing I wanted to do. Unlike previous surgeries, I wasn't allowed to eat or drink. I was beyond feeling hungry, but was definitely weak. A few friends came by and one brought a gift of mint flavored lip balm. I would apply it, lick it off, and apply it again, allowing my taste buds to think I was eating.

The best part of the day was when Brittany walked through the door. Currently living with her husband in Utah,

I wasn't expecting to see her stroll in nonchalantly, flashing her smile and bearing gifts. Plopping a cute stuffed bear on my bed and handing her Dad a sports magazine, she announced her intentions of staying through Friday. She had independently orchestrated her surprise visit including renting a car, and I marveled at how much she had grown since that year following my initial cancer diagnosis. Was she even old enough to rent a car? Where did the time go?

It was a treat having my youngest daughter present with nothing but visiting me on her agenda. She livened up the room with her stories and sunshine. Brittany was a real asset when it came to finding a solution for my unwashed hair. The following day she brought dry shampoo (a product I didn't even know existed), spraying and combing it through my greasy hair, and finishing the look with two French braids. That not only helped disguise the fact I hadn't washed my hair for a week, but kept it off my neck and away from the central line, making it easier to change the dressing and keep the area clean. I was careful not to discuss the possibility of cancer with Brittany, attempting to keep our visit light and carefree. The last thing I wanted was for her to be concerned. Not realizing it at the time, Randy had already told all our children what the doctors were thinking. Since I didn't worry, I assumed no one was anxiously waiting to hear the results from pathology.

That evening I gave Kristy a call just to visit. I could tell she was tense and I soon realized she was extremely worried about my impending diagnosis. For the first time, it dawned on me my family and I were viewing things differently. I shared with Kristy the peace I was experiencing. I could feel her burden being lifted as I told her how calm and unconcerned I was.

Remembering that Julie and her daughter Emilie were planning to leave for Disneyland the next day, I decided to call and share my convictions so nothing would mar their trip.

Julie thanked me profusely and assured me that it helped her to know of the peace I felt.

I had a more difficult time convincing Kimberly, who was experiencing a great deal of anxiety about my situation. If I could get away with it, I would shield her from worry, but it would be worse to not let her know what was happening.

Hanging up from these three conversations, I wondered at my daughters' concern, wishing I didn't have to drag everyone through the worry of cancer again. I hoped my efforts to convince them otherwise had been successful. Even more, I hoped my efforts to convince myself were real.

Wednesday morning brought added strength as I found it easier to get out of bed and walk longer distances. I was still denied food or drink but by this point had surrendered, not having any idea how long this fast would last. A nutritionist came by to visit, informing me what I should eat as soon as I could eat. None of it sounded very appetizing.

I thought back on our drive to Sedona and the resolutions Randy and I had made. I wanted to lose ten pounds. Check. I think I accomplished that, but not in the way I had planned.

It was mid-morning when Dr. Deyden waltzed into my room. I had never seen him so animated and cheerful. Grinning from ear to ear, he announced, "It's not cancer!"

He went on to explain he received the preliminary reports from pathology and the lymph nodes as well as the affected bowel were benign. They were still waiting the results of a stain but this report was indeed wonderful news. As I watched Dr. Deyden express his relief my first thought was, "You really believed it might be cancer?" I marveled at my lack of concern. Was it denial, or was I being naïve? I like to think I had actually accomplished my resolve to not let the fear of cancer control my life. As Dr. Deyden and Randy celebrated the good news, I smiled in wonderment at the scene.

My surgeon's next topic of discussion was recovery. He asked if I had experienced any gas or movement in my abdomen. Knowing my answer determined when I would get to eat, I was sad to give a negative report. He reiterated the importance of not taking even a tiny sip of water and encouraged me to walk often. As quickly as he entered my room, he was gone, leaving Randy and I to rejoice in the happy news he brought.

As each day in the hospital passed, my healing accelerated. I was finally able to tolerate a liquid diet, graduating to soft foods. Five days after surgery, I was released from the hospital to complete my recovery at home. All the nurses and doctors were exceptional, but I thought as I was wheeled out into the sunshine, "I want to get as far away from here as possible and forget this nightmare." I was never so grateful to walk into familiar surroundings, sleep in my comfortable bed, and not be connected to tubes.

Recovering at home, I had plenty of time to begin the process of making sense of the past two weeks. I felt like there were so many unanswered questions. What caused the initial pain in my lower abdomen? Can enlarged lymph nodes generate such extreme pain? Why didn't a blockage show up on the first two CT scans, and was there even a blockage? Was any of this related to the final findings and the removal of a section of my small intestine? If it wasn't cancer, what was attacking the wall of my intestine?

Several weeks after being released from the hospital I had a conversation with Dr. Polowy and I asked him this very question. Being as puzzled as Dr. Deyden he remarked, "I don't know what it was. We all feared it was cancer, and when it wasn't, we had no answers." The medical field, although scientific, cannot always explain what happens in our bodies. Sometimes things occur outside our realm of understanding and we count these occasions as miracles.

I believe in a God of miracles. I feel my doctors were guided to find the problem and remove it, and God took it from there. Besides being physically healed, the greater miracle was the emotional healing that took place as I finally handed my life over to my Heavenly Father and allowed His will to be done. I was willing to do whatever God wanted, even if it meant walking down the cancer road again. I literally placed my life in His hands, and I feel that was what He wanted me to learn.

Knowing that I have more time on this earth, having been spared additional grueling treatments for cancer, is a solemn responsibility. I awake each day, thankful for the chance to be with loved ones, to serve others, and enjoy living. There is more I must accomplish, more to learn, and a need for some fine-tuning. I don't want to waste a moment of this precious gift of time.

Rounding the final bend of my cancer road, I took a moment to turn and look where I had been. Were there potholes I wished I had skirted around, or boulders I would remove instead of climb? What choices would I make differently? What would I do again?

One of the huge boulders I climbed was teaching school. A common comment I heard from family and friends was, "I can't believe you taught school during your treatments." I never considered not continuing with my job. My major concern was how to make it work.

Attempting to fulfill my role as a teacher during treatments was the most difficult part of my journey. There were many times I questioned this choice and it caused a lot of physical and emotional stress. I remember one morning backing out of the driveway on my way to school and seeing my next-door neighbor, a retired nurse, beginning her morning walk. I was instantly filled with envy as I pictured her returning for a relaxing breakfast, a few household chores to fulfill, or leave undone according to her own desires. I saw her reading a book, or visiting casually on the phone with family. She had control of her day. My day was filled with the possibility of unknown struggles that come when working with children, long hours of standing, teaching new concepts, and a trip at the end of the day to receive more chemo. Right then, I hated my life.

There were many days I seriously wondered how I would get up and face another day in the classroom. I was so exhausted by the end of the year I questioned my own wisdom in teaching during such a challenging time. Then I thought back on what those children did for me that year. I remembered the hugs, eyes full of hope, engaging smiles, and their trust in me to provide them with their scholastic, physical, and emotional needs. I was able to see past the exhausting, frustrating days to the joyful, happy moments that made it all worthwhile and kept me going day after day: reading them my favorite books and sharing insights about the literature we studied, watching incubated duck eggs hatch into the cutest creatures possible, feeding caterpillars until they tripled in size and watching them emerge from a chrysalis to become a beautiful butterfly, and wondering how our Elf on the Shelf found a new place to hide each day before Christmas vacation. I loved my students, and they were the antidote that countered the effects of chemotherapy. They gave me a reason to get out of bed and think of something nobler than my own challenging situation. Sometimes the most difficult things in our lives turn out to be what is best for us.

One of my most complex choices was deciding not to continue taking Arimidex following my chemotherapy. Someday I may have to face the consequence of that decision, but as each year passes and I am cancer free, I rejoice in my ability to move easily, keep up with my energetic family, and pursue the things I love. My reaction to this drug led me down paths I didn't like but my choice to discontinue it will always be in the back of my mind. It was a risk, but one I would take again to enjoy the quality of life I desperately want.

What about breast reconstruction? So far, I have not regretted skipping multiple surgeries to have two artificial breasts. The way I see it, they are not much different from the silicone prostheses I have, except mine have the advantage of being removable, giving me freedom from the extra weight. The door is always open for breast reconstruction, but as the years go by, I don't see me opting for elective surgery, especially when I'm happy with the way I am.

There is one thing I would change if I had to walk this road again. I waited far too long to connect with other cancer patients. It took me awhile to even accept the fact I was one. I remember receiving phone calls from a representative of the American Cancer Society and wondered why she would be calling me. I didn't understand why a social worker came into my hospital room after my mastectomy.

Not realizing I needed assistance and support along the way, I gave up opportunities to make my journey less distressing and lonesome. After I found the breast cancer support group and figured out there were people out there who were also travelling a similar path, I could finally begin the process of acceptance and healing. I have made remarkable friends and, together, we have come to understand and cope with the many effects that are attached to a cancer diagnosis.

Even though each cancer patient faces a unique experience, there are common threads that bind us together. We all know the gut wrenching fear resulting from the words, "It is cancer". We feel the uncertainty of the path ahead. Each cancer patient must plot his course, change it when necessary, and forge through pain and trials. I once believed that the finish line was the end of treatment, but I now know that, for me, it was conquering fear.

Seven years after being diagnosed with breast cancer, I have finally relinquished the need to be in control of all outcomes, trusting in God who is in charge. This process was not an easy one for me. My personal journey had many detours and bumps and I acknowledge the possibility of more to come. What has changed is not the road, but my ability to navigate it with faith, not fear. It took me a long time to achieve this, but the prize doesn't go to the first one to arrive at the finish line, but to everyone who eventually reaches it.

The Danish Christian philosopher Soren Kierkegaard wisely counseled, "Life can only be understood backwards; but it must be lived forwards." Writing my story has made me look backwards and in the process, I have discovered myself. Having done so, I must now press on, always cognizant of the lessons I've learned and what my journey with cancer has helped me become. To fully live is to embrace each day with love, enthusiasm, and faith in God. My story is far from over, but the effects of cancer no longer dictate my every move. I did more than just survive. I found meaning in the suffering, hope in the storm, and faith in the road that stretches ahead. It is time to live forward.

And once the storm is over you won't remember how you made it through, how you managed to survive. You won't even be sure, in fact, whether the storm is really over. But one thing is certain. When you come out of the storm you won't be the same person who walked in. That's what this storm's all about.

— Haruki Murakami, *Kafka on the Shore*

# BOOK CLUB DISCUSSION QUESTIONS

1. At the beginning of her journey, Claudia formed a cancer "file" in her mind where she shoved all information she couldn't handle. How was this helpful in the beginning? How was it detrimental in the long run? What methods of coping with difficult information or circumstances have you used?

2. What is something you have feared in your life? How did you finally overcome it?

3. Claudia's mom was the last to find out she had cancer. How do you think that made her mom feel? Have you ever hesitated to share something with a loved one and why?

4. Claudia chose to continue her job of teaching school during her surgery and subsequent treatments. From your point of view, what benefits did she reap from this choice, and what were the negative consequences of her decision?

5. What are the difficult questions you would discuss with your loved ones if you were faced with a life-threatening illness?

6. For Claudia, choosing the right surgeon and oncologist made all the difference in her experience. Share a time when your choice of a doctor or professional proved to be advantageous or detrimental.

7. Hair loss was a big issue for Claudia. In what ways would you handle it differently than she did, or what would you do the same?

8. Have you ever adopted a theme, quote, or scripture to help you through a difficult situation? What was it? In what ways did Claudia's theme "Undaunted" help her?

9. During some of her darkest moments, Claudia felt the presence of unseen angels which she attributed to being her family that had gone on before. Have you ever experienced this? How did you feel and how did it help you?

10. Addictions can come in all shapes: bad habits, technology, medication, drugs, to name a few. Have you ever had to deal with an addiction in yourself or a loved one? How did it affect your life and how did you overcome it or help a loved one overcome one?

11. After her treatments ended, Claudia finally sought out a breast cancer support group. Have you ever joined a support group and in what ways did it help you? How do you think Claudia's journey would have been different if she had sought a support group earlier on her cancer road?

12. What factors do you think contributed to bringing Claudia to the point where she finally trusted in God and put her life in His hands? How did this trust change her response when faced with another cancer scare?

# ACKNOWLEDGEMENTS

Surviving cancer and writing this book were not two separate events. One facilitated the other. I wrote because I survived, and I survived because I wrote. Neither surviving nor writing was accomplished alone.

My team of doctors and nurses were the key players in my fight to physically survive cancer. They are my heroes and I'm forever grateful for their medical expertise and exceptional care. Dr. Polowy led the team with skill and compassion. I trusted and looked to him many times for counsel and reassurance. I had a hard time letting go and returning to my primary care physician when the time came to phase out. For several years following my final chemotherapy treatments, I usually called his office when something new would develop, always concerned cancer might be returning. He was patient with my reluctance to let go, never rushed me at appointments, and he listened. That last thing is very important. To be a compassionate listener and treat patients like people, not statistics, is something to look for in choosing a doctor. It isn't often you find a skilled surgeon like Dr. Deyden who also demonstrated so much kindness and consideration for his patients. Both specialists made all the difference in my long physical journey.

Emotional survival was accomplished with a team of family members, close friends, and those I met along the way. I was required to lead this team. I'm afraid that initially, I wasn't a very good leader. Surviving cancer emotionally was a grief process and the time eventually came for me to face it head on. I was never alone in my efforts, but the final result was all up to me.

How fortunate I was to have a devoted husband that loved and cared so deeply throughout my cancer journey. Randy is the only one who witnessed me at my worst, physically and mentally, yet he loved unconditionally. Trying to remain strong, he kept his sorrows and worries to himself. That had to be hard.

I am blessed with six amazing children who supported me, each in their own individual way. Thank you, Julie, Kimberly, Kristy, Autumn, Doug, and Brittany. I couldn't be more grateful for the strength you provided and the encouragement and prayers you offered. I offer special acknowledgement to my youngest daughter Brittany who experienced a much different senior year of high school than most youth, demonstrating courage and faith as she shared my daily battle. Thanks to my sweet mother who prayed, called daily, and loved as only a mother can.

So many people contributed in various ways to make this book possible. Thanks to my family who offered encouragement and to Randy who persevered and made the first edits. Grammatically, he was a tough editor, and we had many conversations where I would defend my literary license versus the rules of syntax. He is the methodical one of the two of us which gives balance to our marriage. Thank you Sarah Hinze, Laura Lofgren, Sue Marshall and Diann Knipp, for your interest in reading my first drafts. Your encouragement kept me writing and striving for improvement. I thank my son-in-law James for being my technical support and teacher and providing many hours to help set up my website. Thanks to Dr. Polowy and my son Doug for helping with the medical terms. I'm not holding them responsible for all medical references, as you must remember that the book is written from the patient's point of view, which I admit can sometimes be skewed.

When I discovered my editor, Kathy Fowkes, I knew I had found the one for the job. Initially, we visited over the phone before I handed her my baby. It was frightening to release my manuscript to a professional, having no idea how it would be received, but a necessary step in moving forward. Thank you, Kathy, for not mincing words, being honest, and helping me achieve the writer within. You pushed me to dig even deeper, making my story what it was meant to be. With your insights, suggestions, and valued time and skills, I was able to make my dream become a reality. Thank you for believing in me, for your encouragement and enthusiasm, and for being my partner in this process. And a special thank you to your "staff", including Rachael Fowkes, who designed the perfect flourish for adding a personal touch to my journal and dedication pages.

One of my biggest concerns was coming up with an appropriate cover. Not only was it important to catch the eyes of potential readers, but I wanted it to depict my cancer journey. When the cover was being designed, I had not met the talented artist that was creating it, yet it was as if she knew me and understood my journey. When I saw the cover for the first time, I knew it was right in every way—the colors, lighting, style, and voice. Thank you, Abigail Fowkes, for creating an inspiring cover that says with a brush what I feel in my heart.

My book mentions many of my friends, all who impacted my journey in countless ways. Thank you, Monica Germaine and Lauri Benson, for the many rides to the hospital, doctor, and lab appointments, and always being available to listen. Other friends I would like to thank are Cindy Seeley, Julie Woods, Mack and Rachel Fenn, Janis Thornton, and Rich and Michelle Dinsdale. Countless others helped with rides, bringing meals, sending cards, flowers and gifts, visiting and providing encouraging words. I can't begin to list all those who impacted my journey and made me feel loved.

Many have said they didn't know how I continued teaching school while enduring chemotherapy. I didn't do it alone. Thank you, Lori Allen, for the hours you devoted to be my right-hand teacher. You were always willing to step in at a moment's notice and I never worried with you there to take care of my little flock.

Thank you, Sue Marshall, for your patience with my many absences and for not looking too carefully at my inability to measure up that year. Thank you, Peggy O'Neill, for sacrificing personal time to help me pull the year together, and for your constant support and friendship. I am grateful to the Hale Elementary staff for the gifts, cards, kind words, and for cheering me on every single day. What a year that was. And thanks to my second-grade students and their parents who remained confident in my ability to keep on teaching, despite my limitations.

What can I say that appropriately expresses my love for my cancer survival friends whose insights and examples contributed to my journey and this book? Everyone needs someone who has walked the same path; with whom they can share what is hard to express to those on the sidelines. There were many that touched my life, but thanks to Shawna Banovich, Denise Griffin, and Marianne Hobbs who have stayed close. You made the journey laughable, bearable, and almost worth it.

Most importantly, and above all, I acknowledge my Heavenly Father as being a key participant in my recovery and in writing this book. I know that God is aware of each one of us, and loves us individually. He knows our names and He knows our struggles. Sometimes He heals, and sometimes He has other plans for us. I am certain that God knows what we need to learn and experience in life in order to reach our potential. I discovered that trusting in Him and accepting our Savior's atonement was the formula in overcoming my fears and finding peace in my journey.

When I was diagnosed with cancer, I never imagined I would be writing a book about my journey. The decision to help others with a cancer diagnosis, along with the need to look within and process my complex feelings spurred me forward. A project this big could never be accomplished alone, and so I extend my love and gratitude to all those who impacted my journey and to those who helped me share it.

# CONTACT THE AUTHOR

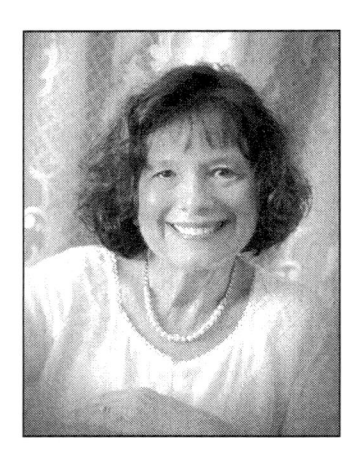

Have a question or comment? I'd love to hear from you!
Please email me at:
cabretzing@gmail.com

Visit my online photo album of my cancer journey:
www.thecancereffect.com

Available for speaking engagements

If you enjoyed this book or received value from it in any way, would you be kind enough to leave a review on Amazon? A sentence or two can make all the difference. Thank you very, very much!

Printed in Great Britain
by Amazon